DIAGNOSTIC PICTURE TESTS IN

INJURY IN SPORT

J. G. P. Williams

MD, MSc, FRCS, FRCP
Medical Director,
Farnham Park Rehabilitation Centre
Consultant in Rehabilitation Medicine,
Wexham Park Hospital, Slough
Civil Consultant in Rehabilitation Medicine, Royal Navy

Wolfe Medical Publications Ltd

8.50

Titles in this series, published or being developed, include:

Diagnostic Picture Tests in Paediatrics
Picture Tests in Human Anatomy
Diagnostic Picture Tests in Oral Medicine
Diagnostic Picture Tests in Orthopaedics
Diagnostic Picture Tests in Infectious Diseases
Diagnostic Picture Tests in Dermatology
Diagnostic Picture Tests in Rheumatology
Diagnostic Picture Tests in Obstetrics/Gynaecology
Diagnostic Picture Tests in Clinical Neurology
Diagnostic Picture Tests in Ophthalmology
Diagnostic Picture Tests in Surgery
Diagnostic Picture Tests in General Medicine

Copyright © J. G. P. Williams, 1988
Published by Wolfe Medical Publications Ltd. 1988
Printed by BPCC Hazell Books Ltd, Aylesbury, England
Reprinted 1991
ISBN 0 7234 0928 5

QT260 WIL

For a full list of Wolfe Medical Atlases, plus
forthcoming titles and details of our surgical,
dental and veterinary Atlases, please write to
Wolfe Medical Publications Limited,
2-16 Torrington Place,
London WC1E 7LT

Preface

There are no such things as 'sports injuries' — only injuries, some of which occur in sport. Many occur in other walks of life as well but some tend to be peculiar to sport, because the mechanisms of their causes are not commonly found in other activities.

This selection of questions and answers presents a number of common injuries and conditions which are used as examplars for the redefinition of specific principles of diagnosis or management. Also included are a number of rarities and unusual presentations to test the ingenuity and deductive skill of the reader and some examples of methods of diagnosis and treatment, further to focus interest in the management as well as diagnosis of these cases.

It is hoped that the collection will be stimulating, instructive and entertaining.

Acknowledgements

During the preparation of this book I had to rely on several colleagues for material, specifically radiological material, and I acknowledge with thanks the help of Roderick Grant, Peter Dovey, Ennis Giordani and David Edwards.

I am also grateful to the clinical photographers at Wexham Park Hospital, Mrs Tyler and Mr Griffin, and at King Edward VII Hospital, Miss Bannister, for their assistance.

for
Sally,
Stephen, Philippa and David
— as always

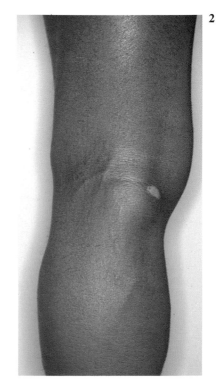

1 A patient injured his finger slip fielding at cricket.
(a) What is the nature of the injury?
(b) How is it treated?

2 A patient has a swelling behind the knee.
(a) What is it?
(b) How is it treated?

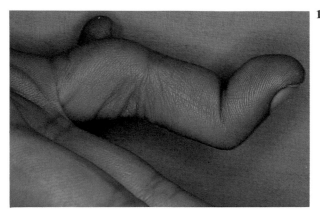

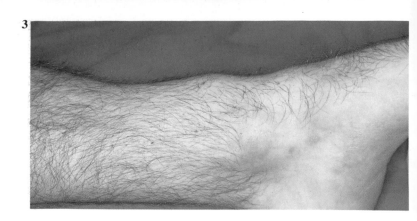

3 A runner had pain over the dorsum of the foot for some months before the onset of swelling.
(a) What is the condition?
(b) How is it treated?

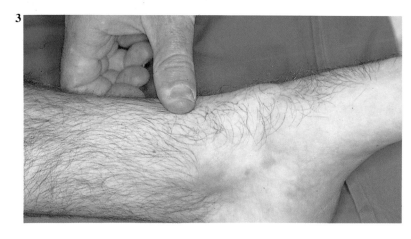

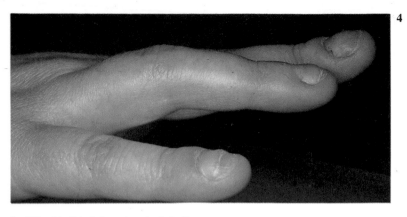

4 What is this injury in a judoka?

5 A patient was struck on the inside of the thigh by a field hockey ball.
(a) What is the condition?
(b) What are the complications?
(c) How is it treated?

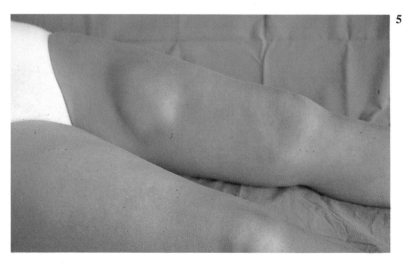

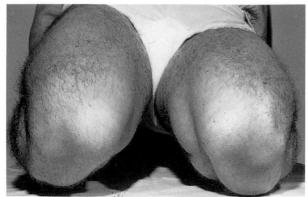

6 A footballer sustained a partial tear of the right quadriceps (rectus femoris). He became unable to squat on his haunches.
(a) What is the reason?
(b) How is it treated?

7 What is this lesion in a patient with no history of trauma complaining of pain in the knee on exercise?

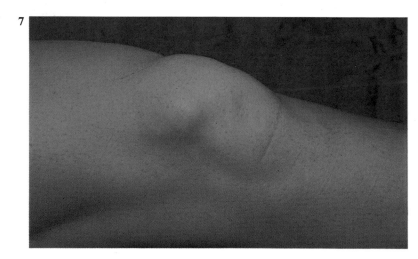

8 What is this lesion in a patient complaining of intermittent pain, swelling and difficulty in extending the knee following a twisting injury while playing football?

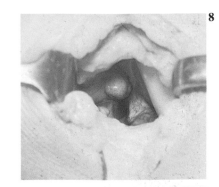

9 A patient complained of pain in the shoulder and difficulty with swimming.
(a) How is the lesion caused?
(b) What is it?
(c) What is its management and prognosis?

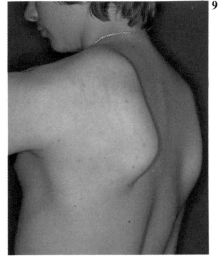

10 An Achilles tendon displayed at operation. What is the painful lesion demonstrated?

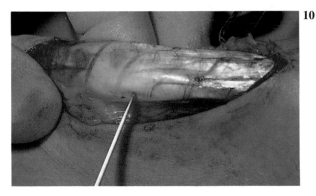

11 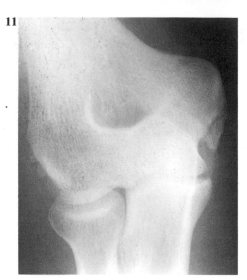 What is this condition causing pain in the elbow in a left-handed tennis player?

12 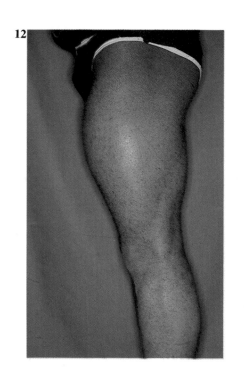 A young man complained of the sudden onset of pain in his left thigh while training.
(a) What is the condition?
(b) How is it managed?

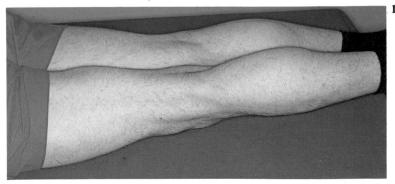

13 A patient is unable to extend his left knee. What is the cause?

14 A patient injured his knee playing football in a collision with the goalkeeper. The knee does not look normal. What is the injury?

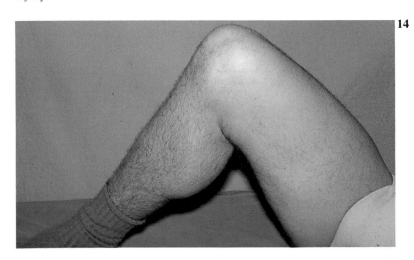

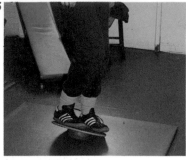

15 (a) What is this apparatus?
(b) For what is it used?

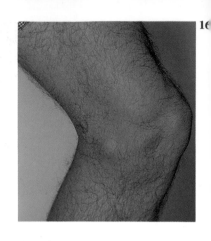

16 A patient with a painful swelling on the medial side of the left knee. What is it?

17 Arthroscopic view of the knee of a footballer who complained of persistent discomfort and swelling in the knee. There was no significant previous history of injury and no other significant signs. What is the diagnosis?

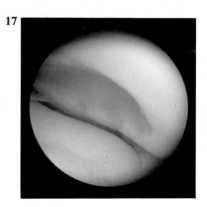

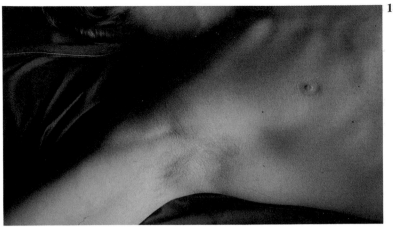

18 A patient complained of persistent pain in the front of the right shoulder, particularly on attempted abduction and external rotation. The onset of symptoms followed a failed tackle while playing rugby.
(a) What is the condition?
(b) How is it treated?

19 A little gymnast complained of severe pain in the back over a period of 4 years. She had been diagnosed as having 'growing pains' and little had been offered in the way of treatment.
(a) What is the condition?
(b) What is its significance?
(c) How is it managed?

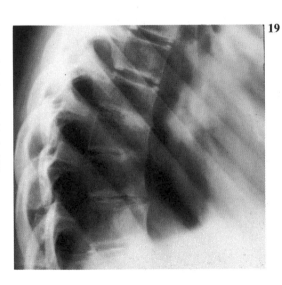

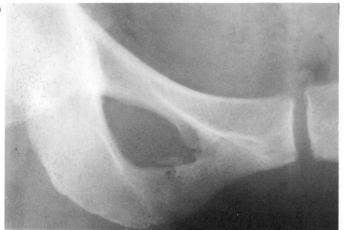

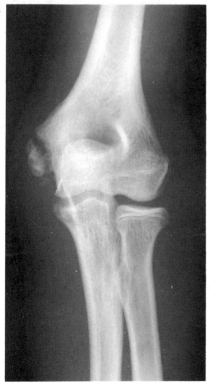

20 A patient complained of pain in the right groin, associated with heavy training for fell running.
(a) What is the condition?
(b) What is the differential diagnosis?

21 A young tennis player complained of pain on the inner side of the elbow.
(a) What is the diagnosis?
(b) How is it managed?

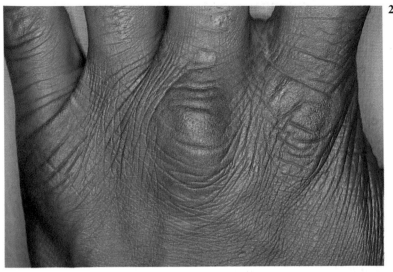

22 A professional boxer complained of pain over the dorsum of the second metacarpophalangeal joint.
(a) What is the lesion?
(b) How is it treated?

23 A junior county table tennis player complained of pain and swelling in the right trapezius after striking her bat on the under edge of the back of the table while trying to make a shot.
(a) What is the condition?
(b) How is it managed?

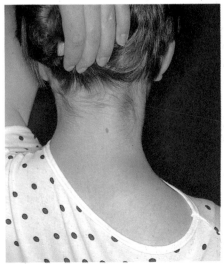

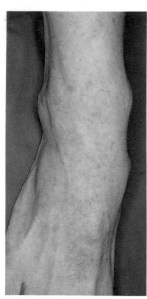

24 A patient complained of pain and swelling on the dorsum of the ankle during exercise. What is its significance?

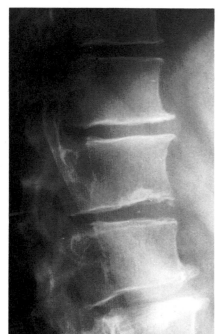

25 Radiograph of lumbar spondylosis in an individual who has been an enthusiastic athlete all his life. What is the significance of the shape of the vertebral bodies?

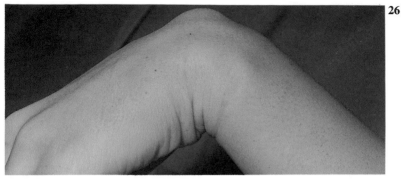

26 (a) What is this swelling on the dorsum of the wrist?
(b) What is its significance?
(c) How is it treated?

27 (a) What is this condition?
(b) Is it significant in sport?

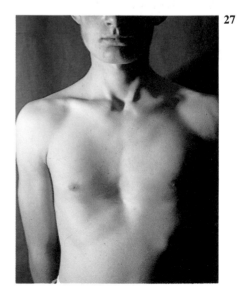

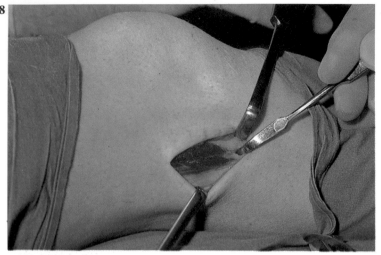

28 A rugby player complained of swelling and discomfort at the outer side of the knee. Is this appearance at operation normal?

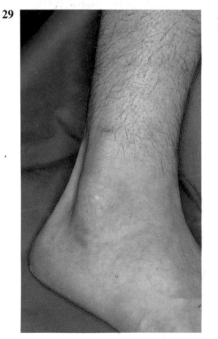

29 (a) What is this condition?
(b) How is it treated?

30 (a) What is this condition?
(b) What is its significance?
(c) How is it treated?

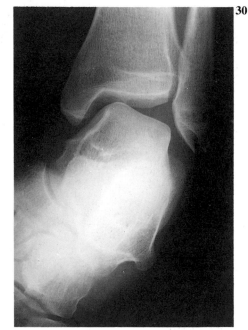

31 A left-handed squash player complained of discomfort in the wrist and difficulty in playing his shots. Clinical examination revealed no obvious abnormality of the wrist. What is the cause of his problem?

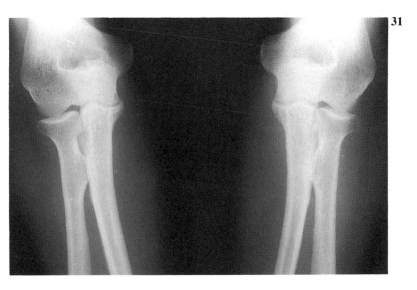

32 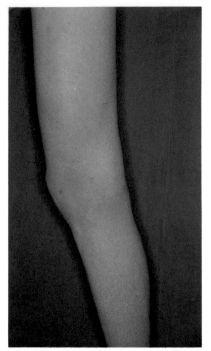 A junior international athlete complained of pain and swelling on the outer side of the left knee, particularly after training. As shown, the swelling is diffuse, extending from the level of the upper pole of the patella down below the level of the head of the fibula.
(a) What is the condition?
(b) How is it treated?

33 A patient injured the proximal phalanx of his middle finger at judo. He presented some months later with persistent pain and swelling; no fracture was visible on radiographic examination. What is the management?

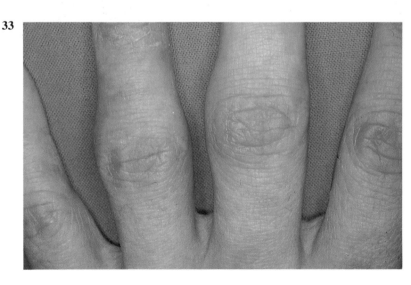

34 (a) What is this condition?
(b) What is its particular significance in terms of sport?

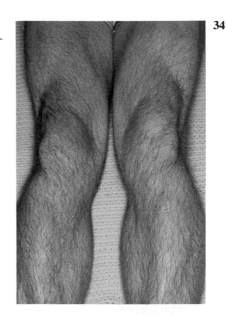

35 A patient complained of pain and exquisite tenderness over the anterior aspect of the shin following a kick while playing football. What is the differential diagnosis?

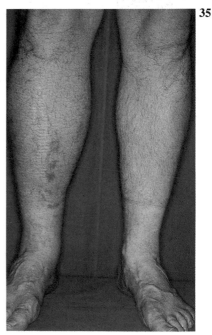

36

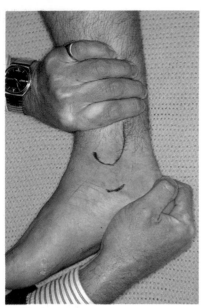

36 What sign is being elicited here in a patient with a history of recurrent sprain of the lateral ligament of the ankle?

37 A patient complained of a sudden onset of pain in the upper arm while attempting to curl with a heavy bar-bell.
(a) What is the condition?
(b) How is it treated?

37

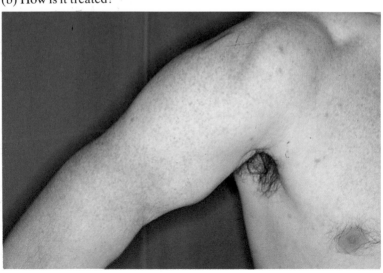

38 A young footballer complained of pain in the knee on exercise.
(a) What is the diagnosis?
(b) What are the complications?

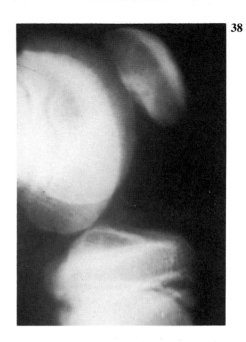

39 A patient complained of gradual onset of pain in the shin on running.
(a) What is the diagnosis?
(b) What is the most significant complication?

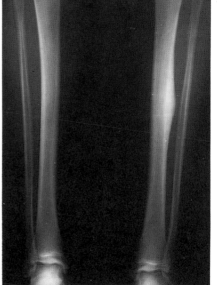

40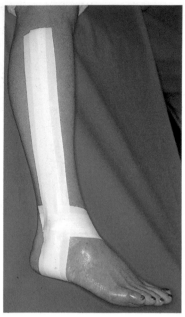

40 (a) What is the purpose of this strapping?
(b) How is it used?
(c) For what condition?

41 A runner complained of a pain in the region of the Achilles tendon. What is the diagnosis?

41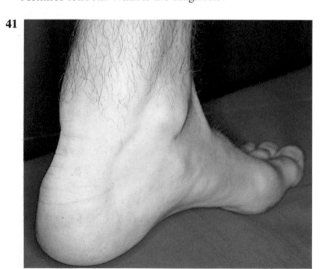

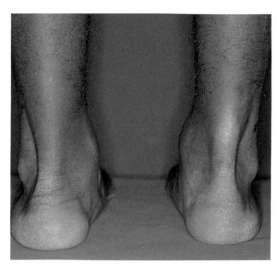

42 What does this photograph show?

43 A patient complained of pain in the hip following a wrench while out running cross-country. What is the lesion?

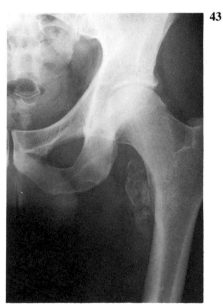

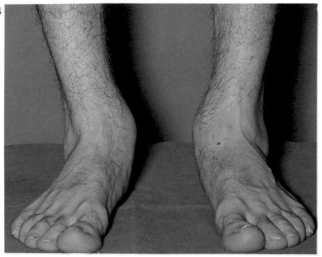

44 What is this condition in a marathon (fun) runner with sore legs?

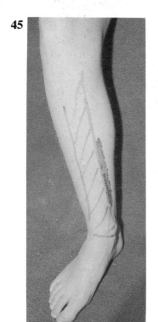

45 A patient complained of pain along the medial border of the tibia in the site indicated. What is the diagnosis?

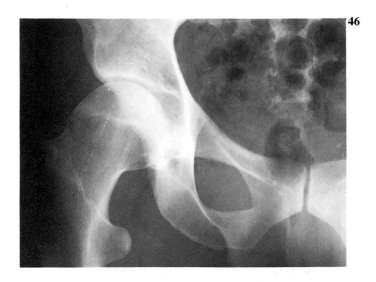

46 (a) What conditions are illustrated?
(b) What is the significance of the line drawn through the head and neck of the femur?

47 A tennis player complained of pain in the chest wall after serving. What is the condition?

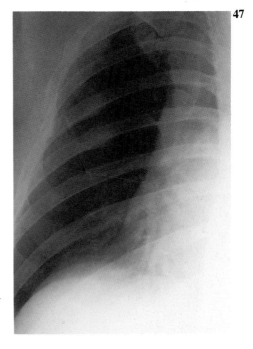

48

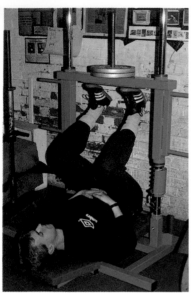

48 (a) What is this apparatus?
(b) How is it used?

49

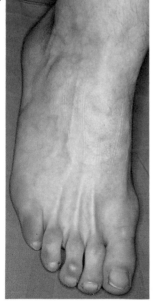

49 What problems is this foot causing?

50 A squash player with no history of injury. What is the condition?

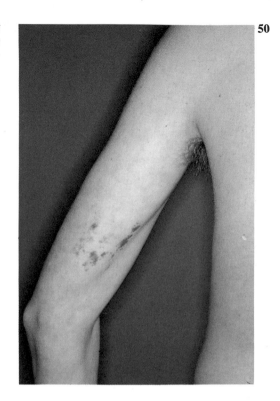

51 What common problem of runners is exhibited here?

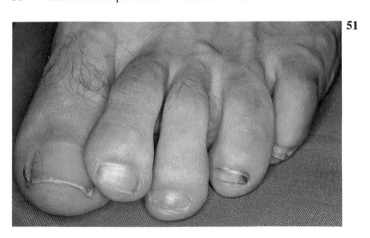

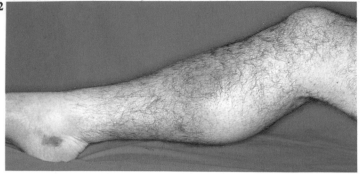

52 A patient complained of a sudden onset of pain in the left calf while running.
(a) What is the diagnosis?
(b) What is it not?

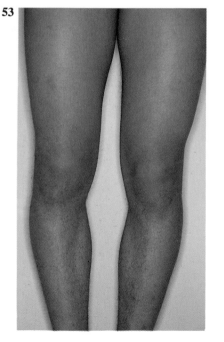

53 (a) What obvious differences are there between these two legs?
(b) What is the significance?

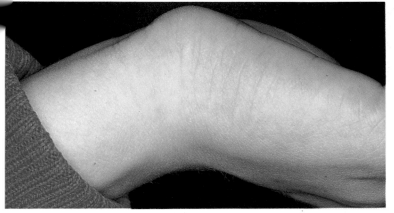

54 A polo player complained of pain in the hand, at the base of the wrist. He was acutely tender over the ulnar border of the wrist on the volar surface. What is the condition?

55 (a) What is this condition?
(b) What is its significance in sporting terms?

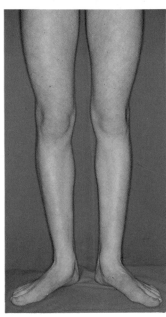

56

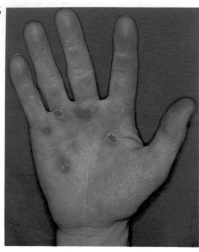

56 A simple well-recognised overuse injury—but how is it best treated?

57

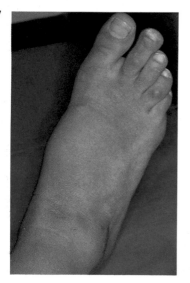

57 A patient injured her foot in a gymnastic accident when landing from a vault and was unable to bear weight. What are the possible diagnoses?

58 Following an old injury, a patient was unable to the extend the elbow fully and the distal end of the humerus was palpably distorted. What common complication may be expected?

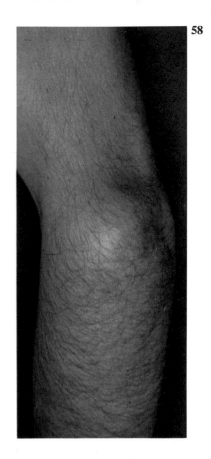

59 (a) What is this condition?
(b) How may it most rapidly be treated?

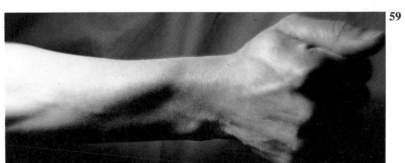

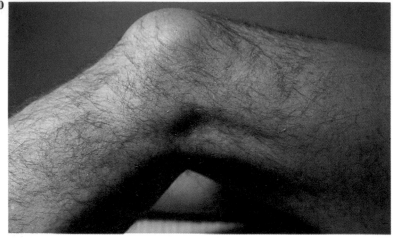

60 A runner complained of pain on the lateral aspect of the knee, particularly when running. There was no significant local tenderness. What condition is indicated here?

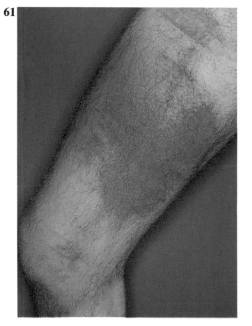

61 (a) What is this condition?

(b) What is its significance in a patient with a history of a muscle tear?

(c) Why does it look layered?

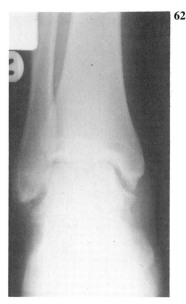

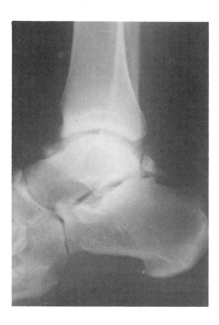

62 What conditions are demonstrated on these radiographs?

63 Radiograph of a young gymnast who fell from the beam and continued to complain of pain in the elbow. What is the diagnosis?

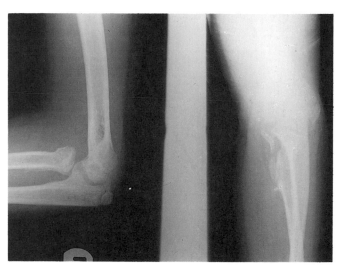

64

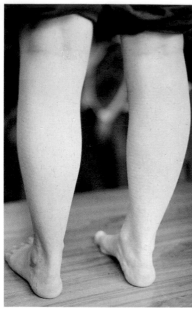

64 With what group of conditions is this configuration of the lower leg associated?

65 What pathology is illustrated?

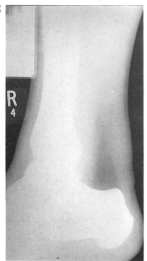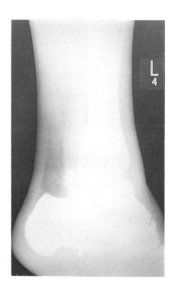

66 A middle-aged woman took part in the London marathon and subsequently complained of pain in the thigh. What is the diagnosis?

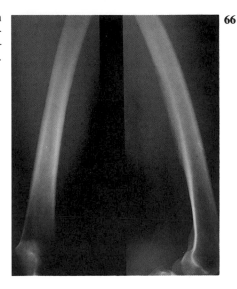

67 A field hockey player complained of pain in the wrist during movement. What structural abnormality is demonstrated?

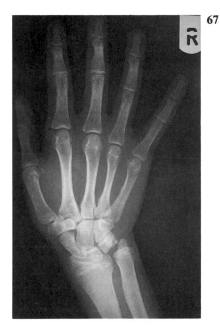

68

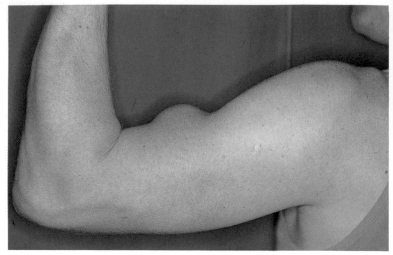

68 (a) What is this condition?
(b) How is it treated?

69 A patient received a blow on the upper arm in attempting a tackle while playing rugby. He subsequently complained of pain and stiffness in the elbow. What is the condition?

69

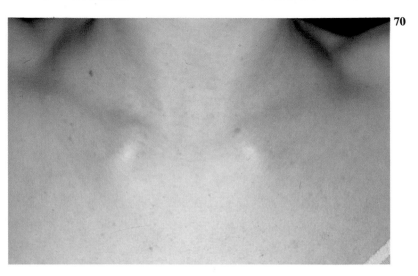

70 A young javelin thrower complained of pain, of gradual onset, at the inner end of the right clavicle. What is the condition?

71 A patient complained of low back pain after weight-training.
(a) What clinical sign is present?
(b) What is its cause?

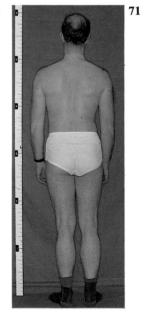

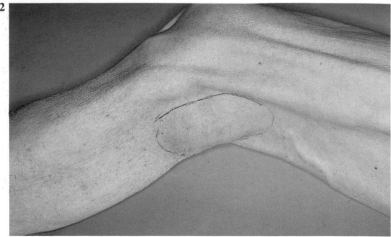

72 (a) What structure is dramatically demonstrated here in the leg of a veteran marathon runner?
(b) What is the lesion outlined?

73 Radiograph of a soccer goalkeeper who sustained a blow on the front of the elbow while saving the ball at the foot of another player.
(a) What is the condition?
(b) How is it treated?

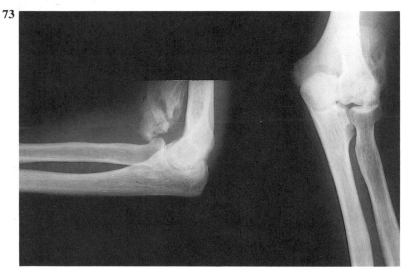

74 A junior international rugby player complained of pain in the elbow, particularly when trying to throw a long pass. What does the radiograph show?

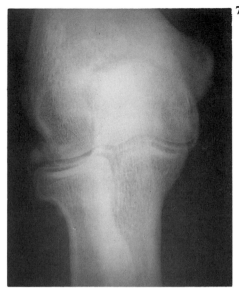

75 A patient developed progressively increasing pain in the right wrist. There was no history of trauma.
(a) What does this radiograph show?
(b) What is the most likely cause of this condition?

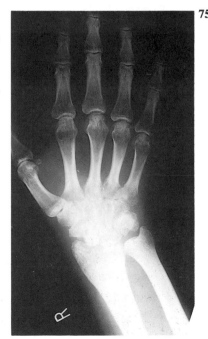

76 A patient complained of pain in the knee when playing football and taking other exercise.
(a) What is the condition?
(b) What is its significance?
(c) How may it be treated?

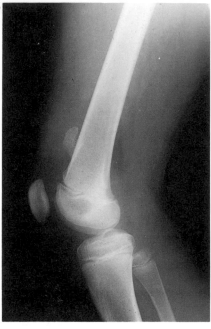

77 A tennis player complained of pain in the right shoulder on movement.
(a) What is the condition?
(b) How is it treated?

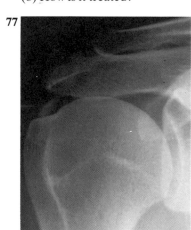 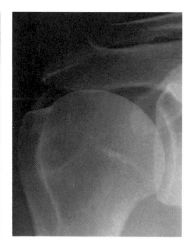

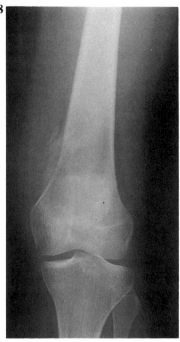

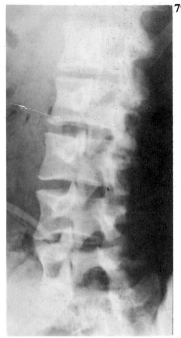

78 A patient complained of knee pain with exercise, of gradually increasing severity. What is the diagnosis?

79 What is this condition, presenting as low back pain in a young pole-vaulter?

80 A golfer presented with anterior knee pain and fullness in the antero-medial aspect of the knee joint. At operation this extrasynovial tumour was removed from the knee joint deep and medial to the patellar tendon. What is it?

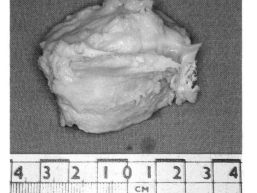

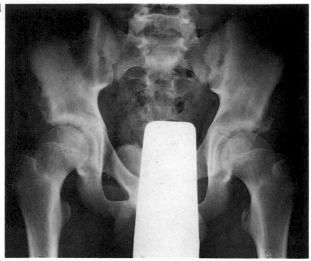

81 A patient complained of pain above the hip on exercise. What is the condition?

82 What does this radiograph of an injured footballer's knee show?

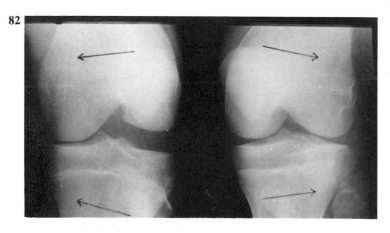

44

83 (a) What is this condition?
(b) How is it caused?
(c) How is it treated?

83

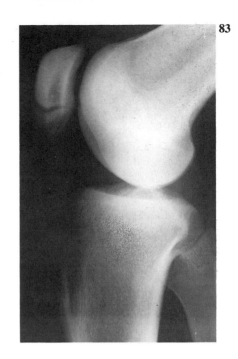

84 A young footballer complained of gradually increasing pain over the lateral aspect of the ankle while running or exercising. What diagnosis should be considered?

84

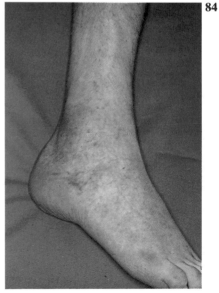

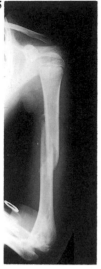
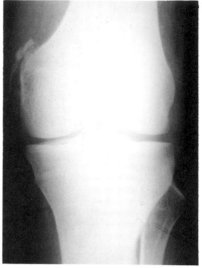

85 A young gymnast fell while vaulting and sustained a spiral fracture of the humerus. What is the major problem in cases of this type?

86 (a) What is this condition?
(b) What is its significance?

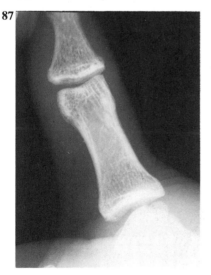

87 This injury of the thumb occurred in an international boxer.
(a) What is the condition?
(b) How is it treated?
(c) How may it be prevented?

88 (a) What is this condition?
(b) How may it be exacerbated in the young sportsperson?

88

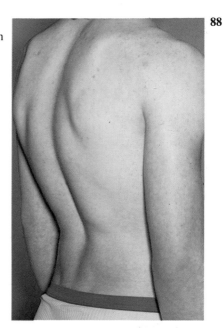

89 This radiograph was reported as 'normal' as there is no obvious bony abnormality.
(a) Is there any abnormality?
(b) If so, what is it?

89

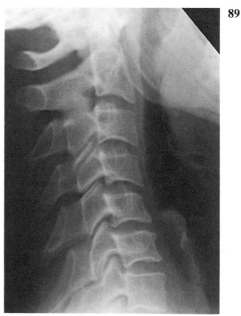

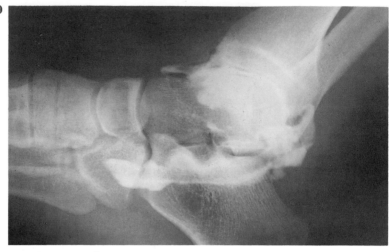

90 (a) What does this radiograph demonstrate?
(b) What is its significance?

91 (a) What is this condition in a young gymnast following a fall from a vaulting horse?
(b) What is its significance?

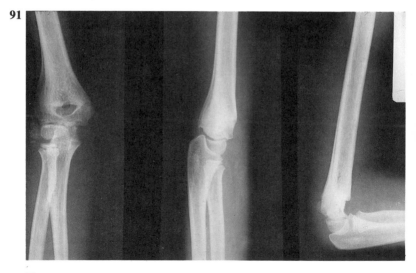

92 A young footballer complained of pain in the heel.
(a) What is this condition?
(b) How is it managed?

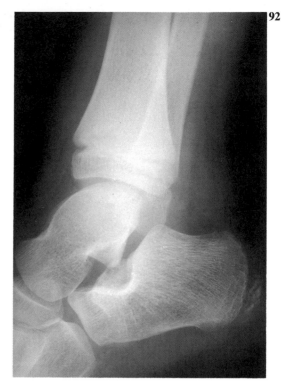

93 What pathologies are demonstrated?

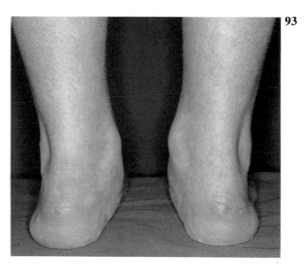

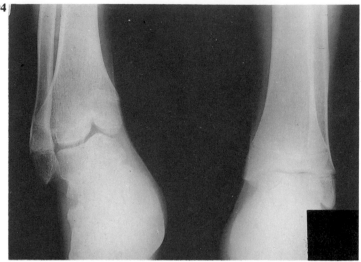

94 Anteroposterior radiograph of the ankle of a young footballer. What is the cause of the distortion?

95 A rugby player complained of pain in the shoulder after tackling. There was no history of specific injury. The pain had gradually become worse.
(a) What is the diagnosis?
(b) What is the treatment?

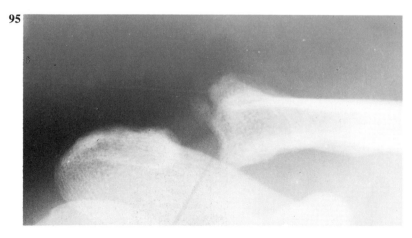

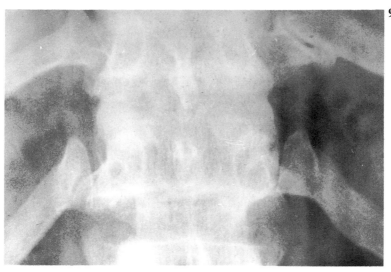

96 A patient complained of lower thoracic and upper abdominal pain while playing golf.
(a) What is the condition?
(b) How is it treated?

97 A young athlete complained of pain at the lower pole of the patella. What is the condition?

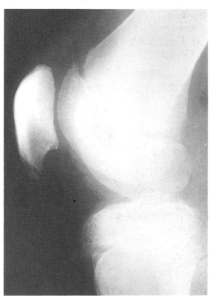

98

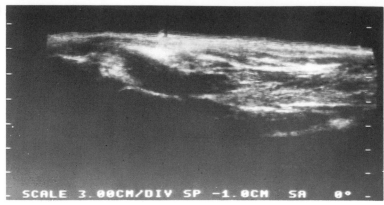

98 A footballer complained of pain in the groin when running. Clinically there was some fullness below the inguinal ligament. What is this investigation, and what does it show?

99

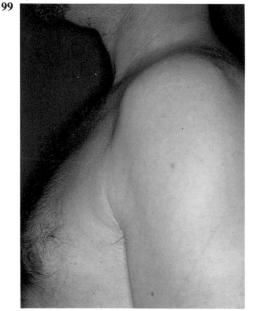

99 A patient was a keen, left-handed, tennis player and complained of pain in the left shoulder.
(a) What clinical sign is shown?
(b) What is the diagnosis?

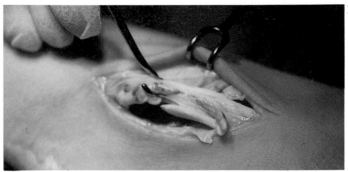

100 A gymnast complained of pain in the left lower leg above and behind the medial malleolus. The pain came on suddenly following a twist at gymnastics, and the patient presented with tenderness above and behind the medial malleolus and a fiercely pronating foot. This is the operative finding. What is the condition?

101 (a) What is this condition?
(b) How may it be treated?

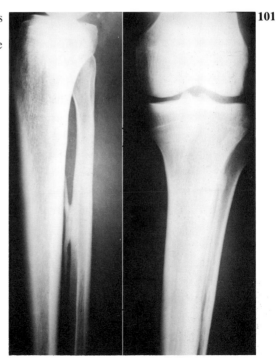

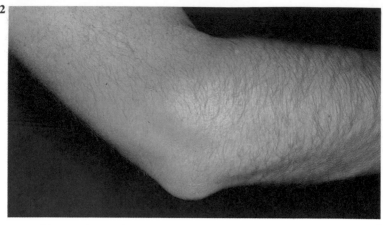

102 (a) What is this condition?
(b) In what sports does it occur?
(c) What can be done (i) to prevent and (ii) to treat it?

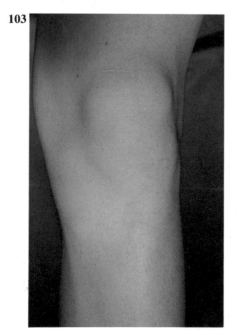

103 (a) What is this condition in a swimmer?
(b) How may it be caused?
(c) How may it be treated?

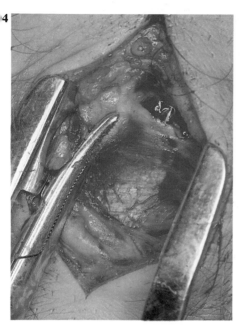

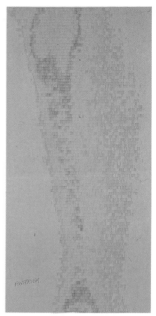

104 What is this condition affecting the patella tendon?

105 Radionuclide scan of the upper tibia in a middle-distance runner who complained of pain. What is the differential diagnosis?

107 (a) What is this apparatus?
(b) What is its use?

106 What is this finding?

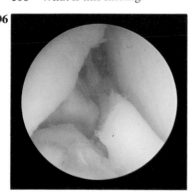

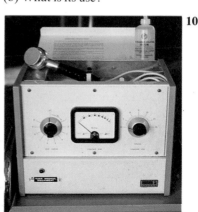

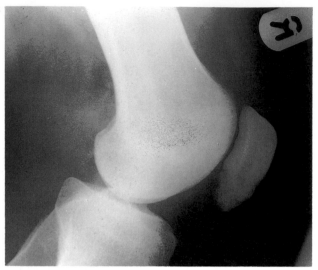

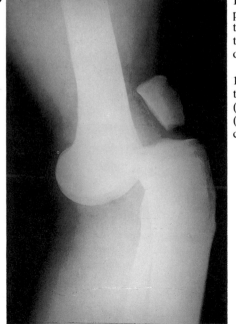

108 A footballer complained of pain in the front of the knee at the lower pole of the patella. What is the condition?

109 (a) What is this condition?
(b) How is it treated?
(c) What are the complications?

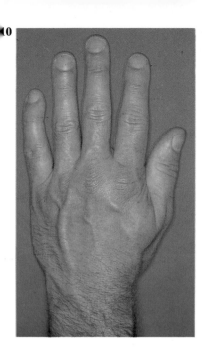

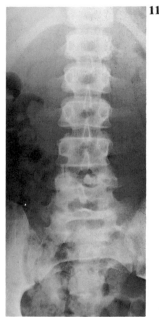

110 A golfer complained of pain in the hands gripping his club and of early morning stiffness. What is the diagnosis?

111 Radiograph of the spine of a young gymnast who complained of pain during training.
(a) What is the condition?
(b) What is its significance?
(c) How may it be treated?

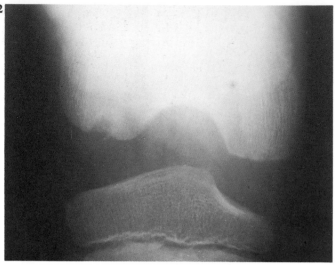

112 What condition is depicted in this radiograph of a young athlete's knee?

113 A long-distance runner complained of pain at the back of the heel.
(a) What is the condition?
(b) How is it treated?

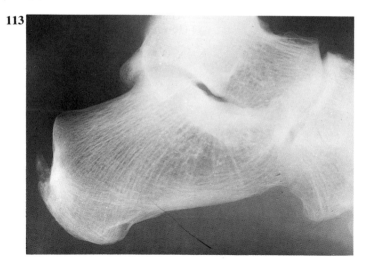

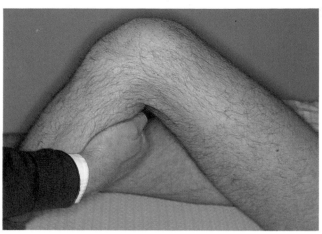

114 (a) What sign is depicted?
(b) What care must be taken in interpreting it?

115 A footballer complained of pain in the little toe after an awkward kick. What is the treatment?

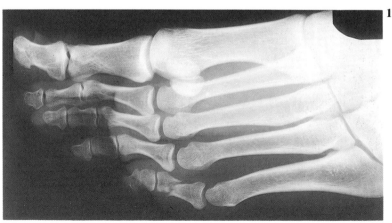

59

116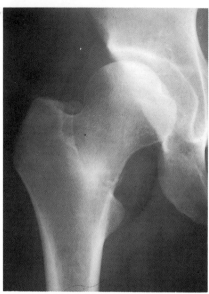

A patient complained of persistent pain in the hip when running. What is the diagnosis?

117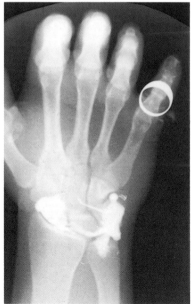

(a) What is this investigation?
(b) What does it demonstrate?

118 This county field hockey player complained of difficulty in breathing on severe exercise.
(a) What is the diagnosis?
(b) What is the appropriate treatment?

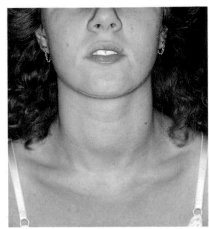

119 A patient complained of a pain in the left sternoclavicular joint following a tackle while playing rugby.
(a) What is the condition?
(b) How is it treated?

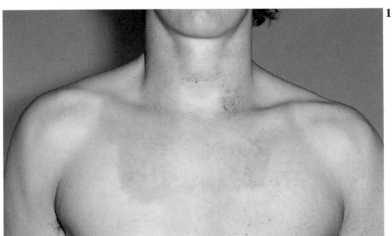

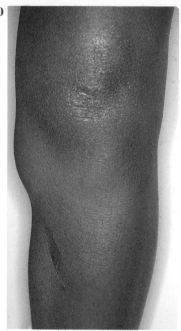

120 A patient complained of pain and swelling over the medial aspect of the tibia, interfering with his play in basketball. The condition had developed insidiously and was characterised by a soft tender mass over the medial aspect of the tibia, with some evidence of thickening of the bone deep to it. What is the cause?

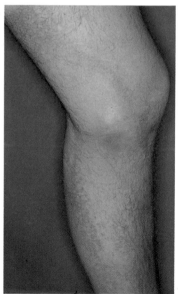

121 What is this painful swelling on the medial side of the knee following a kick playing football?

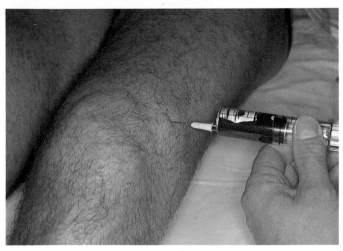

122 (a) What is this procedure?
(b) When should it be carried out?

123 (a) What is this condition?
(b) What is it not?
(c) How should it be treated?

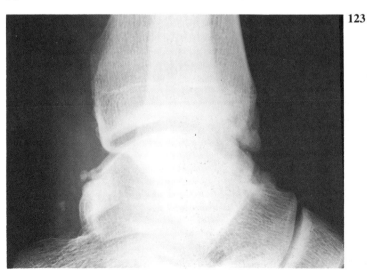

124

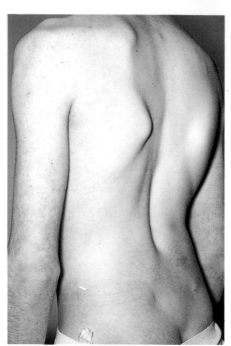

124 What is the cause of the 'step' in this patient's back, and what is its significance?

125

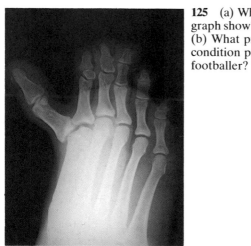

125 (a) What does this radiograph show?
(b) What problems does this condition pose for a talented footballer?

126 (a) What is wrong with this patient?
(b) What advice should be given regarding sport?

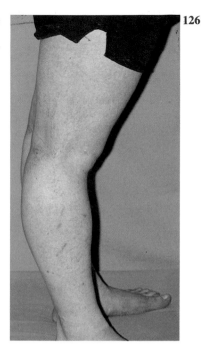

127 (a) What is this condition?
(b) To what is the appearance due?

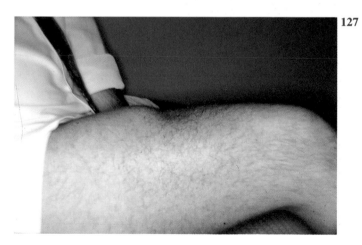

128

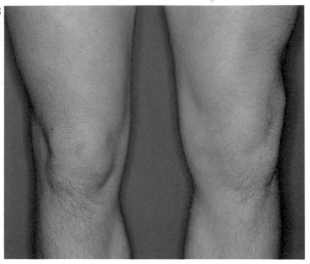

128 A patient sustained a wrench of the knee while playing football. It swelled very rapidly and he was unable to continue playing. What is the cause?

129

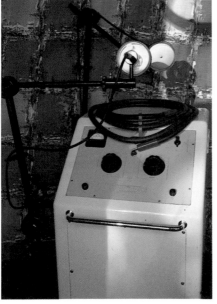

129 (a) What is this apparatus?
(b) For what is it used?

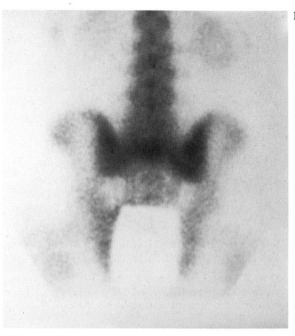

130 (a) What is this investigation?
(b) What is demonstrated?

131 (a) What is this condition?
(b) How should it be treated?

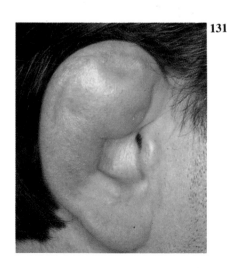

132

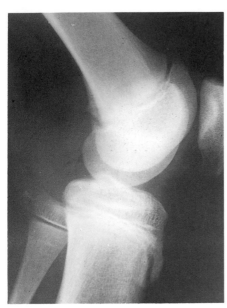

132 (a) What is this condition?
(b) What is its significance?
(c) How should it be treated?

133

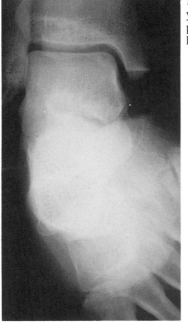

133 Radiograph of the ankle of a young gymnast who complained of pain after exercise, with no previous history of injury. What does it show?

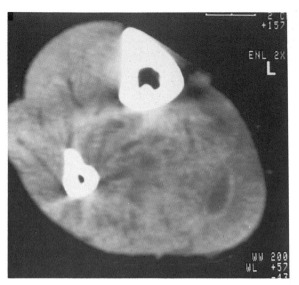

134 A patient complained of pain and stiffness in the calf following what felt like a blow on the back of the leg while playing racketball.
(a) What is the investigation?
(b) What does it show?

135 (a) What does this radiograph show?
(b) What is its significance?

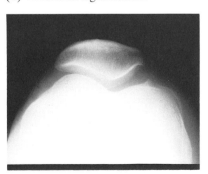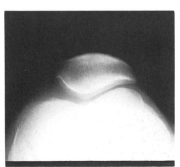

69

136

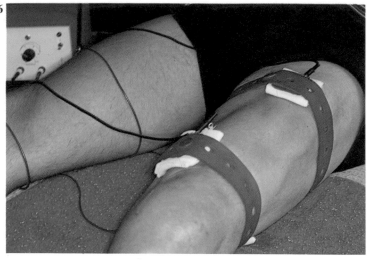

136 (a) What is this apparatus?
(b) What is its use?

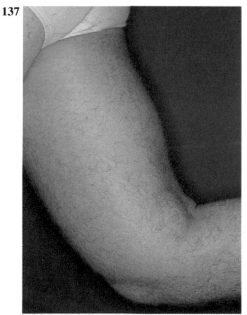

137 A patient deve-
loped a painful swelling
on resisted active flex-
ion of the knee. What is
the condition?

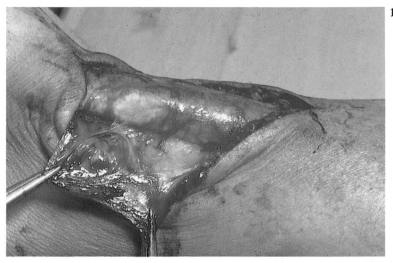

138 What is this condition in the Achilles tendon?

139 A patient complained of persistent giving way of his knee associated with anterior knee pain. What physical sign is demonstrated?

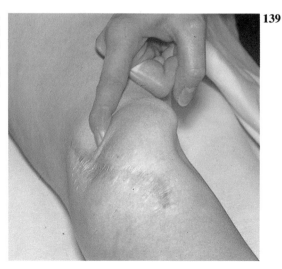

140

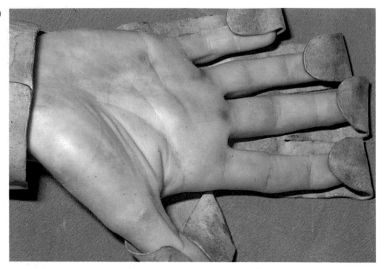

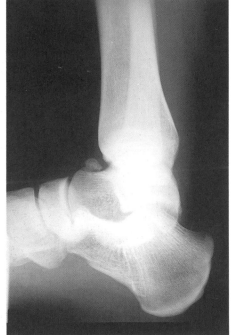

140 A fencer complained of pain in the hand and jamming of the middle finger in flexion. What is the cause?

141 (a) What does this radiograph of a jogger's ankle show?
(b) How is it treated?

142 (a) What is this investigation in a footballer with a history of pain and locking in the knee?
(b) What does it demonstrate?

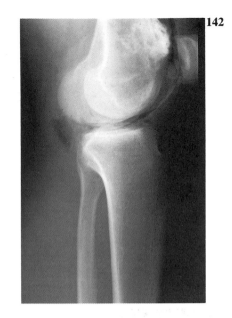

143 (a) What is this condition?
(b) What problems does it create?
(c) How does it present?

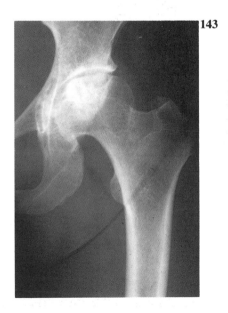

144 A young gymnast complained of pain behind the ankle after gymnastics.
(a) What condition is demonstrated in this radiograph?
(b) How may it be managed?

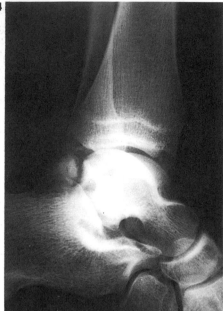

145 A marathon runner complained of pain in the heel. What is the significance of the radiological findings?

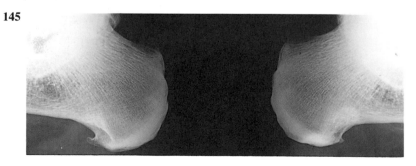

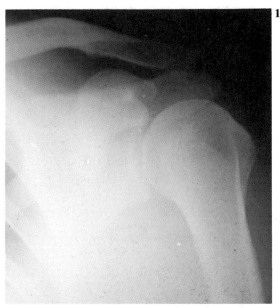

146 (a) What lesion is demonstrated in a football player who has fallen on his shoulder?
(b) How should it be treated?

147 What lesion in an enthusiastic middle-aged jogger is demonstrated?

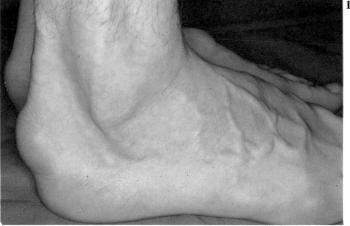

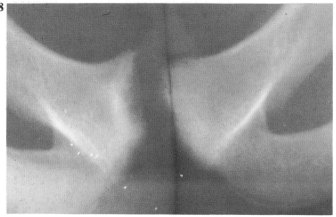

148 A footballer complained of persistent pain and aching in the groin, radiating up to the lower abdomen and down into the left testicle.
(a) What condition is demonstrated?
(b) How is it treated?

149 (a) What condition is demonstrated?
(b) What is its sporting significance?

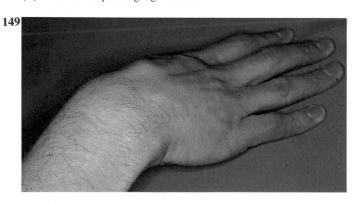

150 The diagnosis is obvious in this radiograph, but what is the pitfall in a case of this kind?

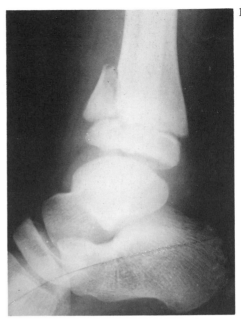

150

151 A patient came off 'second best' in a brawl on the football field.
(a) What are the lesions?
(b) What is their significance?

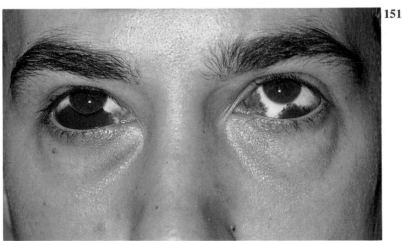

151

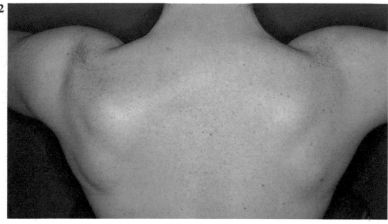

152 A weight-lifter felt a sudden sharp pain in the upper part of the left shoulder. What is the diagnosis?

153 A patient complained of gradual onset of pain in the right groin, interfering with sprinting.
(a) What is the diagnosis?
(b) How is the condition treated?

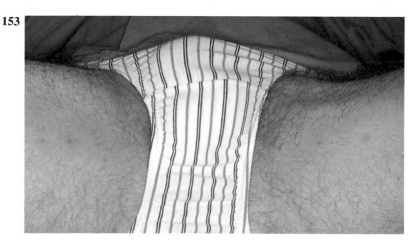

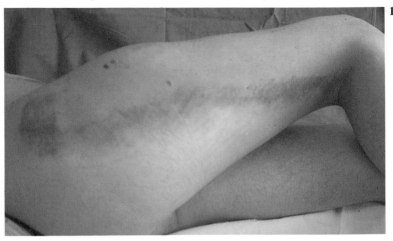

154 A patient slipped and fell on his right side onto a hard ground while playing football. What is the pathology?

155 A patient complained of pain in the dorsum of the wrist while playing squash. What has happened?

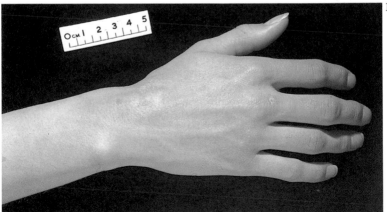

156

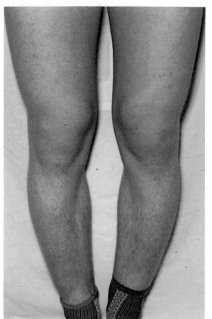

156 (a) What is this condition?
(b) What is its significance in sport?

157 A 14-year-old boy complained for some time of pain at the back of the heel. Playing football, he suddenly developed severe pain and a limp.
(a) What is the diagnosis?
(b) What is the treatment?

157

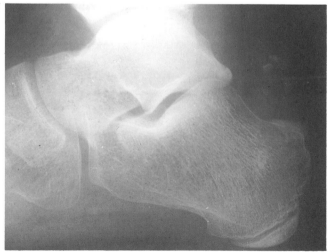

158 A gymnast twisted her ankle landing from a vault.
(a) What is the diagnosis?
(b) What practical problem may such a case present?

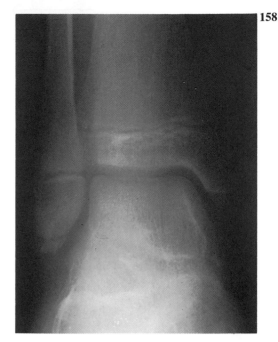

159 A young footballer complained of pain in the hip after a tackle.
(a) What is the diagnosis?
(b) What is the treatment?

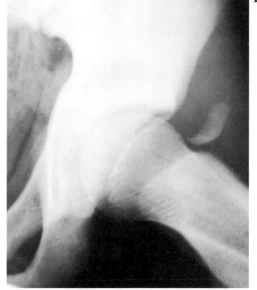

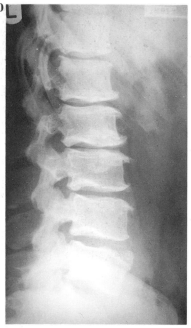 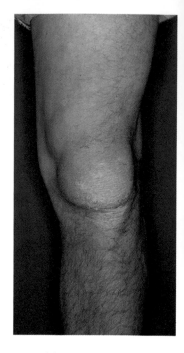

160 (a) What is this condition?
(b) With what sports may it be
particularly connected?

161 (a) What is this condition, and in what sports may it occur?
(b) How should it be treated?

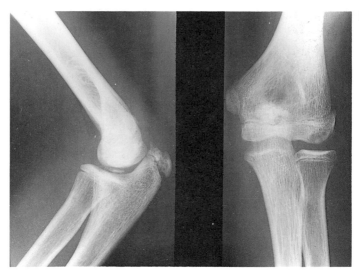

162 A young tennis player complained of pain in the elbow. What is the diagnosis?

163 A patient complained of a painful swelling on the outer side of the knee. What is the diagnosis?

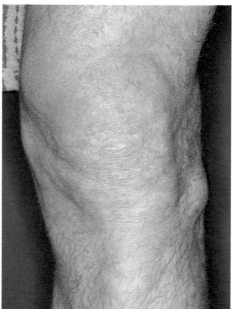

83

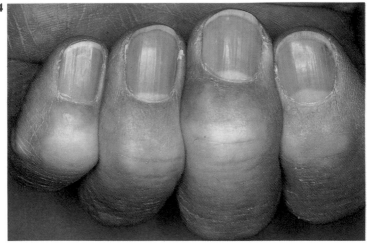

164 A golfer complained of pain in the fingers on gripping his clubs. What is the diagnosis?

165 A squash player felt a sudden bang in the back of the heel while playing. This is the operative finding. What is the diagnosis and management?

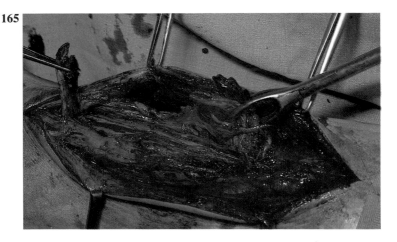

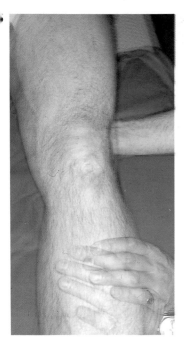 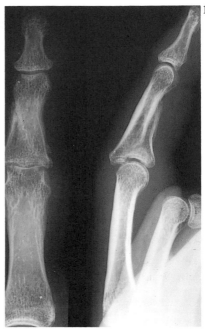

166 What does this double-exposure photograph demonstrate?

167 A patient presented complaining of pain in the finger following an injury while catching a cricket ball.
(a) What is the diagnosis?
(b) What is the management?

168

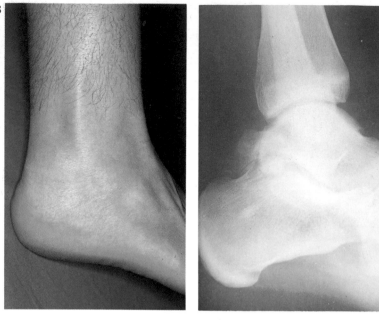

168 A footballer complained of pain and swelling behind and to the lateral side of the ankle. There was no specific history of injury, but ankle joint movements were restricted. What is the diagnosis?

169

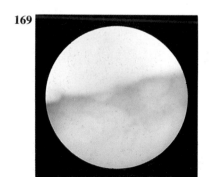

169 (a) What is this condition, seen through the arthroscope?
(b) Is this arthroscopic finding significant?

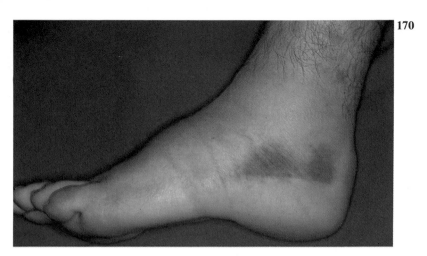

170 What is this condition?

171 What does this radiograph show?

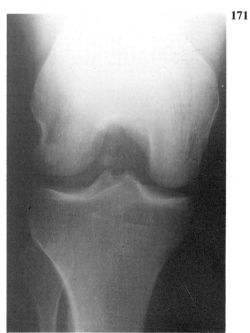

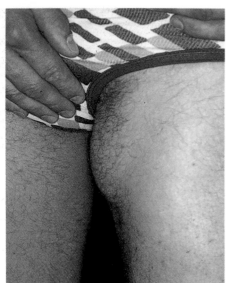

172 A patient complained of sudden onset of pain in the groin while stretching for a tackle when playing football.
(a) What is the diagnosis?
(b) What is the management?

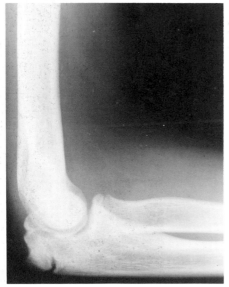

173 A young tennis player complained of pain at the back of the elbow. What is the condition?

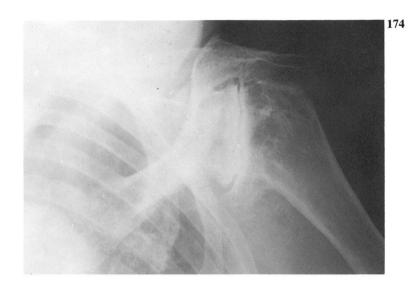

174 (a) What is this condition?
(b) What sports injury predisposes to it?

175 (a) What does this radiograph show?
(b) How should the condition be treated?

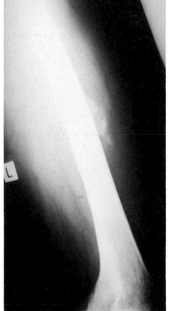

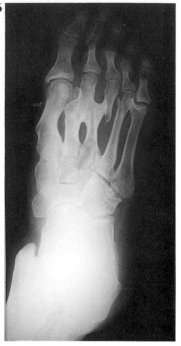

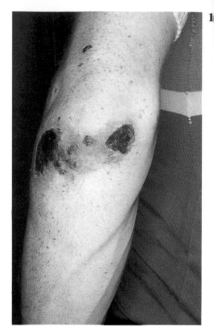

176 A patient sustained an injury to the foot when young, resulting in the deformity demonstrated. What advice can be given to this patient on participation in sport?

177 A cyclist was spilt on to the road in a multiple pile-up in a long-distance road race.
(a) What is the nature of this injury?
(b) What is its particular complication?

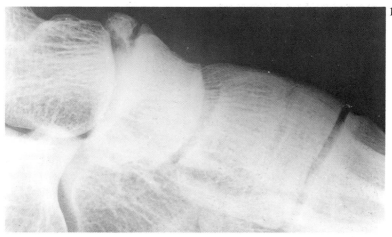

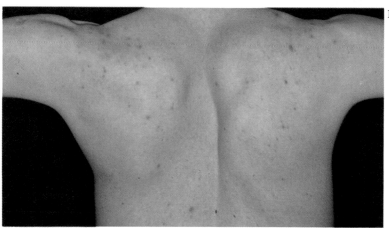

178 Radiograph of the foot of a middle-distance runner who complained of persistence of pain following a twist running cross-country.
(a) What condition is demonstrated?
(b) How may it be treated?

179 A tennis player complained of pain between the shoulders on serving.
(a) What is the obvious clinical feature demonstrated?
(b) What is the most likely diagnosis?

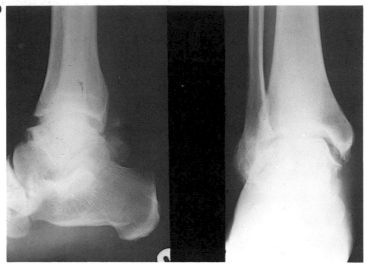

180 A keen footballer: what does the radiograph demonstrate?

181 (a) What is this condition, demonstrated at operation in a middle-distance runner who complained of persistent heel pain? (b) How may it be treated?

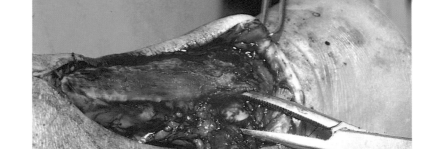

182 (a) What painful condition of the heel commonly seen in long-distance runners is demonstrated?
(b) How should it be treated?

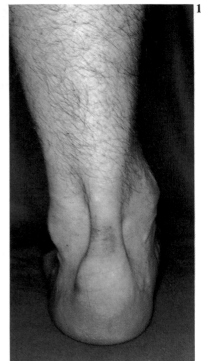

183 (a) What condition is demonstrated in this 400 m runner with a chronic Achilles tendon pain?
(b) What principle does it illustrate?

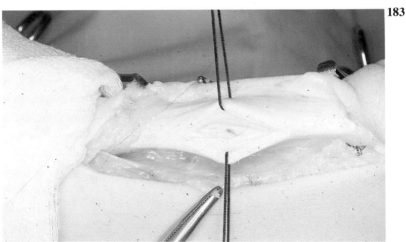

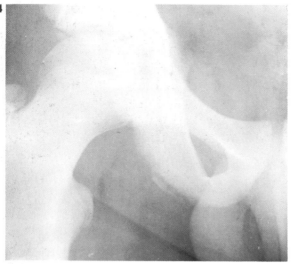

184 An enthusiastic young footballer complained of a sudden onset of pain in the groin while playing. Symptoms persisted in the face of attempts to 'run it off'.
(a) What is the diagnosis?
(b) What is the treatment?

185 A little gymnast complained of pain in the neck following a fall tumbling.
(a) What is the diagnosis?
(b) What is the management?

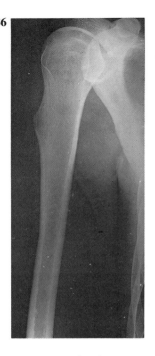
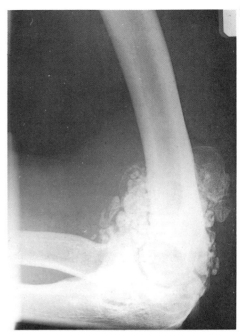

186 A tennis player complained of pain in the upper arm while serving. What is the significance of this radiographic finding?

187 Radiograph of the elbow of a squash rackets player who complained of increasing pain and stiffness in the joint.
(a) What is the diagnosis?
(b) What is the treatment?
(c) What is the prognosis?

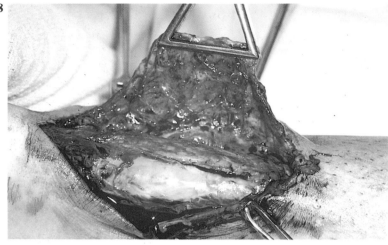

188 A middle-distance runner with a history of persistent Achilles tendon pain who had previously had an exploration of the Achilles tendon. However, his symptoms persisted and re-exploration was required.
(a) What is demonstrated in this operative photograph?
(b) What lesson does it convey?

189 A patient complained of gradual onset of low back pain associated with weight-training. There was no specific history of injury.
(a) Why may this clinical appearance be significant?
(b) What is the most likely cause for the swelling?

190 A patient complained of a pain and throbbing in the front of the leg following a blow while playing field hockey.
(a) What is the likely diagnosis?
(b) How is it treated?

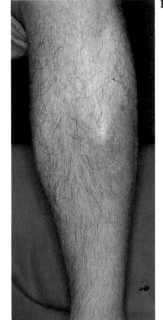

191 A patient complained of persistent pain and instability in the right ankle following a twist playing badminton some weeks previously.
(a) What is the probable diagnosis?
(b) How should it be treated and managed?

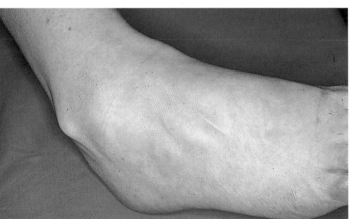

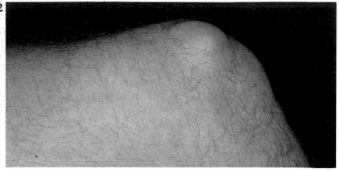

192 A footballer presented with a painless lump on the anterolateral aspect of the right knee that had progressively increased in size. What is the diagnosis?

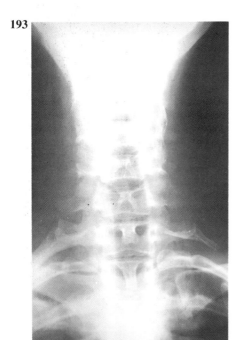

193 A patient complained of pain and tingling in the arm when serving at badminton. What is the probable diagnosis?

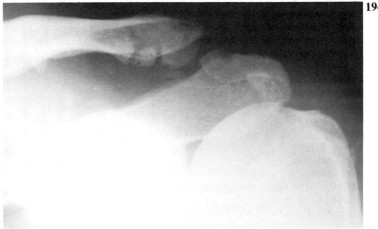

194 Radiograph of the shoulder of a rugby player who fell awkwardly when making a tackle. What clinical abnormalities are demonstrated?

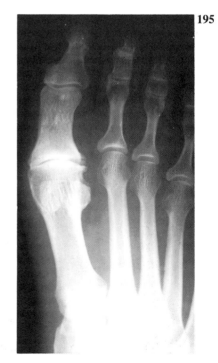

195 A radiograph of the foot of an enthusiastic golfer who complained of pain in the big toe.
(a) What is the condition?
(b) How may it be treated?
(c) What problems may arise?

196

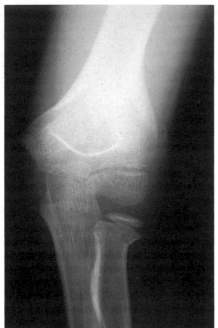

196 A young man fell on his outstretched hand, injuring his right elbow.
(a) What is the diagnosis?
(b) What is the treatment?

197

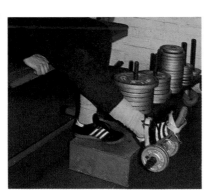

197 What is wrong in this picture?

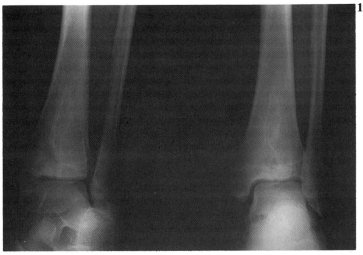

198 A schoolboy developed progressively increasing pain in the ankle doing normal school sport. There was no history of injury. On clinical examination the only finding was a raised skin temperature over the lower tibia. There was no swelling or local tenderness and no limitation of ankle joint mobility. These are the radiograph and scan. What is the diagnosis?

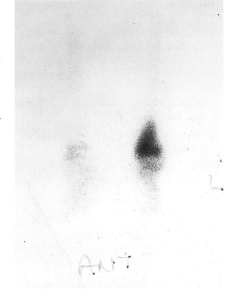

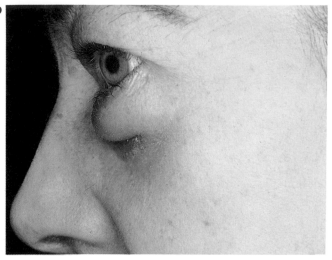

199 A patient received a blow on the face while playing rugby.
(a) What is the diagnosis?
(b) What are the complications?

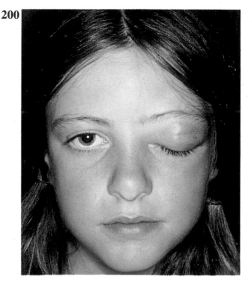

200 A patient was struck in the eye by a ball.
(a) What is the obvious diagnosis?
(b) What other problems may be present?
(c) How should the case be managed?

ANSWERS

1 (a) Mallet finger.
(b) Immobilisation with the proximal interphalangeal joint flexed and the distal interphalangeal joint hyperextended, or by tenodesis.

2 (a) Popliteal cyst. Sometimes wrongly referred to as a Baker's cyst. May be associated with gastrocnemius on the lateral side or semimembranosus on the medial side.
(b) Treatment is expectant. Where the cyst is an embarrassment to activity surgical excision may be carried out, but recurrence is often a problem. Aspiration is not indicated as it leads to chronic inflammation and loculation.

3 (a) This is an effusion into the extensor sheath of the long extensors of the toes following chronic tenosynovitis. The cystic swelling extends both proximal and distal to the extensor retinaculum.
(b) If the presence of the cyst interferes with function then excision is required. Preservation of the extensor retinaculum is not necessary.

4 Boutonniere deformity, with longitudinal splitting of the extensor hood allowing the proximal phalanx to push up between the leaves of the extensor tendon. Treatment requires surgical repair of the extensor hood to correct the deformity, but a perfect result is unusual.

5 (a) Haematoma of the skin and subcutaneous tissues.
(b) It may go on to fatty necrosis in the subcutaneous tissue and intradermal scarring with persistent discomfort and tightness in the skin. The haematoma may liquefy or become infected and encysted.
(c) Primary treatment is application of a pressure bandage and vigorous mobilisation.

6 (a) Loss of extensibility in the muscle, which may be due either to residual chronic inflammatory oedema or a degree of adaptive shortening. In some cases fibrosis in the muscle may cause true tethering.
(b) Treatment is essentially preventive, with early post-injury mobilisation and active stretching of the damaged muscle. A stretch programme is essential and premature resumption of sport should not be permitted, otherwise recurrence is almost inevitable.

7 Bipartite patella. This is a congenital condition often confused with a patellar fracture. The 'fragment' is found almost invariably at the upper and outer quadrant of the patella. It may be thickened and enlarged as in this case, and the undersurface is often malacic.

8 Damage to the alar folds. The menisci and cruciate ligaments are not the only intra-articular soft tissue structures which can be damaged in stress injuries of the knee. The alar fold is pedunculated and may become thick and oedematous as a result of being repeatedly drawn between the joint surfaces, so presenting symptoms similar to internal derangement of the knee due to meniscal tear. In some cases adhesions develop between the alar fold and the intercondylar septum. In established cases the injured margin of the alar fold is damaged frequently and loose bodies may develop in fragments detached from the margin. Treatment is surgical removal.

9 (a) Winging of the scapula due to serratus palsy caused by a virus infection.
(b) Neuralgic amyotrophy.
(c) Treatment is expectant and prognosis is excellent, with full recovery in due time.

10 A well-localised area of tendinitis showing the typical matt grey swollen appearance contrasting dramatically with the glistening appearance of the normal tendon distal to it.

11 Calcification in a chronic medial epicondylitis. Golfer's elbow is relatively common in left-handed tennis players as a result of playing whipped forehand returns. Treatment may be conservative or surgical—in chronic cases the formed bone must be excised and the common flexor origin detached from the medial epicondyle.

12 (a) To all outward appearances this patient had a straightforward quadriceps tear and was initially treated for such. However, swelling in the thigh persisted and became more marked. Ultimately it became clear that this was a malignant tumour (a rhabdomyosarcoma). Haemorrhage into such a lesion can occur with trauma in athletic training.
(b) When in doubt about a lesion of this type ultrasonic scanning will often provide a satisfactory differential diagnosis.

13 Hamstring spasm producing a typical firm swelling in the medial hamstrings on attempting to extend the knee. Following knee injury hamstring spasm is relatively common, and because the patient in such a case is unable to extend the knee fully an incorrect diagnosis of locking may be made.

14 Complete posterior cruciate ligament tear. A soccer goalkeeper falling on the ball at the feet of an on-coming forward may strike the lower leg, driving the tibia backwards in relation to the femoral condyles and causing a posterior cruciate ligament tear. This injury also occurs in American football.

15 (a) A wobble board.
(b) It is most commonly used for rehabilitation following ankle injury. It produces loaded motion in two planes at the ankle joint and is of particular benefit in developing proprioceptive feedback following joint injury.

16 Cystic meniscus. Typically meniscal cysts occur in relation to the lateral meniscus, but they may occur on the medial side.

17 Healing subchondral fracture on the femoral condyle. Fractures of the articular cartilage over a femoral condyle, particularly the medial femoral condyle, are not uncommon in body-contact sports. The actual incident provoking the damage may be slight and unremembered. In the acute phase a definite pit is seen. With time this heals in, giving a shallow crater with rounded margins, as demonstrated here arthroscopically.

18 (a) Partial rupture of the pectoralis major. This condition only became apparent when the shoulder was examined under general anaesthetic with appropriate muscle relaxant.
(b) Excision of the fibrous tissues and vigorous mobilisation to restore extensibility in the muscle.

19 (a) Congenital vertebral fusion (subsequently confirmed by tomography) with osteoarthritic changes in the vertebral joints above and below the site of the block.
(b) Limitation of movement in the spine, due to congenital or acquired fusion, throws excessive stress on the segments of the spine above and below, and may give rise to pain.
(c) Management is by a programme of formal mobilisation together with appropriate supportive muscle exercises so that adequate compensation can be developed during childhood.

20 (a) Stress fracture of the inferior pubic ramus.
(b) The differential diagnosis is from traumatic osteitis pubis, adductor origin strain and obturator hernia.

21 (a) So-called golfer's elbow is common in adult left-handed tennis players. In adolescence, before skeletal maturity (as demonstrated in this case by the presence of the open radial epiphysis), osteochondritis of the bony origin of the muscle is more common than soft tissue damage.
(b) This is an overuse injury requiring management by a period of relative rest.

22 (a) Boxer's knuckle, or adventitious bursa.
(b) Treatment is essentially symptomatic. If severely disabling, excision may be carried out but recurrence is frequent on return to sport.

23 (a) Muscle tear in the trapezius. In table tennis the trapezius acts as a prime mover in elevating the shoulder during the top-spin shot. If this movement is blocked then direct muscle tearing can occur.

(b) Treatment is by a combination of anti-inflammatory medication, physiotherapy and exercise.

24 Low muscle fibre insertion on a tendon is a relatively common cause of symptoms in athletes. The hypertrophy of the muscle fibres consequent on exercise in training causes obstruction either (as in this case) under an extensor retinaculum or at the adit to a tendon sheath.

25 This appearance is relatively common in patients with a history of osteochondritis of the spine in adolescence. Note the slight vertebral wedging and the uneveness of the disc spaces, and evidence of old Schmorl's nodes.

26 (a) A ganglion associated with the inferior radio-ulnar joint.

(b) These are relatively common and cause disability in patients who require full hyperextension in the joint.

(c) Management is by dispersion or, in the intransigent case, by surgical excision.

27 (a) Pectus excavatus. This distortion of the sternum and anterior rib cage is essentially a congenital abnormality.

(b) It may cause problems, partly by reducing the vital capacity of the chest and partly by fixing the chest wall, so reducing respiratory excursion. In severe cases surgical correction may be justified.

28 This patient had an abnormal accessory belly of the biceps femoris. This accessory muscle belly may be the site of 'compartment' symptoms and in established cases a fasciotomy of the overlying tissues may be required to restore comfort.

29 (a) Dislocating or slipping peroneal tendons. In these cases the peroneal tendons come to lie superficial to the lateral malleolus rather than behind it.

(b) In established cases with significant disability reconstruction of the tendon sheaths may be carried out with or without some elevation of the posterior margin of the malleolus.

30 (a) Talar tilt demonstrated by stress radiography. The angle between the upper surface of the talus and the inferior surface of the tibia is greatly increased due to subluxation of the talus in the ankle joint mortice following complete rupture of the lateral ligament of the ankle.

(b) These cases are frequently associated with recurrent sprains and pain, swelling and disability.

(c) Surgical correction may be required.

31 There was no obvious radiological defect at the wrist. However, at the superior radio-ulnar joint there is distortion of the head of the radius, preventing normal rotation of the radius on the articular facet on the ulna. In this case failure of full pronation and supination due to mechanical derangement at the elbow joint produced symptoms at the wrist joint.

32 (a) A cavernous haemangioma. This essentially benign lesion had become relatively large by the time the patient was approaching maturity. The swelling had been present for some time.
(b) Early diagnosis and treatment of cavernous haemangioma by ligature of the feeders prevents the complications that may present with a long-established lesion of this type. In this particular case the haemangioma did not extend into the knee joint, so localised excision and ligature of the feeders was possible.

33 This patient had almost certainly sustained a subluxation of the proximal interphalangeal joint. Following such an injury persistent fusiform swelling is the rule. Treatment is reassurance and active use.

34 (a) Genu valgum or knock-knee.
(b) The patellofemoral joint is particularly at risk in genu valgum because the Q angle (the angle between the line of pull of the quadriceps tendon and the line of pull of the patellar tendon) is increased, thus enhancing the tendency of the patella to ride laterally in the patellofemoral groove when the knee is extended under load. The valgus knee is also more at risk to abduction stresses, resulting in damage to the medial ligament.

35 The soft tissues overlying the anterior border of the tibia are particularly at risk in body-contact sport and a direct blow may lead to haematoma formation with subsequent sepsis and/or cellulitis, or—as in this case—to subperiosteal haematoma.

36 The anterior draw sign. Patients with complete rupture of the anterior bundle of the lateral collateral ligament of the ankle have a positive draw sign, the foot subluxes forwards in relation to the lower leg when rupture is complete. This sign is said to be more specific for complete rupture than is talar tilt.

37 (a) Rupture of the tendon insertion of the biceps brachii.
(b) In most cases surgical repair following this injury gives disappointing results, but it should be attempted if the patient is left with marked loss of ability forcibly to pronate. In most cases, however, only simple mobilisation of the arm and compensatory muscle build-up are required.

38 (a) Osteochondritis dissecans of the patella.
(b) The most important complication is separation of the fragment with loose body formation and locking of the joint.

39 (a) Stress fracture of the tibia. This is relatively common in runners.
(b) If the patient is allowed to continue with activity the crack may progress to a complete fracture. Differential diagnosis is from interosseous hypertension and anterior tibial cortical hypertrophy (pretibial stress syndrome), both of which are also overuse or stress reactions.

40 (a) This is a stirrup strapping.
(b) It is applied to the lateral side of the ankle and the leg overlying the peroneal group of muscles. Such a strap is applied with the foot slightly everted and plantargrade.
(c) In patients who have sustained lateral collateral ankle ligament sprains.

41 A congenital structural abnormality of the triceps surae. The gastrocnemius component was inserted on to the posterior aspect of the calcaneum by a flat band-like tendon. The soleus component was inserted by a direct muscle insertion on to the calcaneum deep to the gastrocnemius component. There was no soleus tendon. Congenital abnormalities can produce symptoms and may cause confusion.

42 Thickening and discoloration around the right Achilles tendon. The loss of pigmentation and the apparent erythema is typical of the effect of previous steroid injection.

43 On first appearances this may appear to be ectopic calcification in the adductors. However, close examination shows that the medial cortex of the femur is eroded. This was in fact a calcifying chondrosarcoma. Haemorrhage into such a lesion or into structures round such a lesion may occur during athletic activity and will often predispose to misdiagnosis. The index of suspicion must be maintained.

44 Mechanically pronating feet associated with tibial torsion. Loss of normal pronation and supination during the stance phase of running due to collapse of the medial ray of the foot produces biomechanical stresses, not only in the foot but also in the leg. Static correction by orthotics should be accompanied by dynamic correction using postural re-education and intrinsic muscle development.

45 Posterior or medial tibial syndrome. This is a form of compartment syndrome characterised by a tearing of the attachment of the fascia overlying the muscles of the medial compartment from the medial border of the tibia. It usually originates in the lower third of the leg, but in an established case the whole of the medial tibial border may be affected. It is a relatively common overuse injury following running on hard ground.

46 (a) Early degenerative joint disease and distortion of the hip joint.
(b) There is a positive tilt deformity characterised by an increased femoral head ratio. This condition is commonly found in patients with traumatic osteitis pubis.

47 Stress fracture of the angle of the rib. Stress fracture at the serratus attachment is not uncommon in tennis players. It is caused by repeated and excessive angulation during the muscle action of serving.

48 (a) Leg press. This is a method of applying load to the extensor muscles of the knee in compression. The weight is captive—that is, its range of movement is clearly defined and controlled and the rest of the patient's bodyweight is taken off the knee joint.
(b) It is a very valuable adjunct for controlled muscle build-up in the knees.

49 Difficulty in obtaining suitable shoes. Callosities on the third, fourth and fifth toes and the bunion over the fifth metatarsal head show evidence of rubbing. Sportspeoples' feet are generally wider than the norm and unless shoes for the chosen sport are available in a number of width fittings problems with pressure and rubbing can be significant.

50 Cavernous haemangioma. It is of little clinical significance unless it is large and invading the underlying soft tissues or joints. In this case the lesion was purely superficial.

51 Subungual haematoma. More commonly the hallux and second toe are affected. Recurrent subungual haematoma with repeated shedding of the nails may lead to distortion of the nail bed and subsequent overgrowth of nail. This is a recognised occupational hazard of long-distance runners.

52 (a) Partial rupture of triceps surae, typically belly of gastrocnemius —in this case the medial head. Treatment in the acute phase is to strap the leg with elastic adhesive strapping from toes to below the knee and to encourage the patient to take as vigorous exercise as possible. This will frequently, albeit painfully, resolve symptoms within a matter of hours.
(b) The condition is *not* rupture of the plantaris longus as was previously described.

53 (a) Quadriceps wasting.
(b) Loss of quadriceps tone and bulk is an almost inevitable concomitant of knee injury. When established it will invariably cause symptoms in the knee to persist. It must in all cases be treated by vigorous quadriceps exercises to restore tone and bulk.

54 Chondromalacia of the pisiform. Damage to the joint between the pisiform and the triquetral is relatively common and may produce symptoms of persistent pain and tenderness. In severe cases treatment by excision of the pisiform is justified.

55 (a) Marked torsion of the tibiae. The plane of the foot is grossly rotated compared with the plane of the knee.
(b) Such patients find great difficulty in running, since the normal mechanism of pronation and supination during the stance phase is distorted. The condition is essentially untreatable, and patients should be directed towards more suitable physical activity—for example fishing!

56 Blisters such as these on hands and feet can, in the acute phase, cause considerable disability. They are readily treated by applying elastic adhesive strapping with the sticky surface directly over the blistered area. No other form of dressing is required. This form of treatment is remarkably comfortable, and because of the exudation from the blistered site the adhesive surface of the strapping does not stick to the blistered areas. It does, however, stick to the surrounding tissues, providing protection. A simple and most effective remedy.

57 Fracture of one of the tarsal bones, particularly the navicular, or, as in this case, subluxation of the midtarsal joint. This injury can occur when the foot is forcibly plantar flexed, as in a bad landing in gymnastics or in a cycling or motorcycling accident.

58 Ulnar neuritis with pain and paraesthesiae down the ulnar border of the hand and, in established cases, diminution of sensation in the ulnar aspect of the ring and the whole of the little finger, possibly together with weakness in the intrinsic muscles of the hand. Ulnar neuritis appears to be more common in patients with distortion of the lower end of the humerus following previous trauma when such patients are physically very active.

59 (a) Extensor tenosynovitis of the wrist affecting the radial extensor tendons—a common complaint in oarsmen and canoeists.
(b) Recent experience has shown that surgical decompression of the extensor pollicis longus and the abductor pollicis brevis muscle bellies allows rapid return to sport.

60 Iliotibial band syndrome. This is a bursitis between the iliotibial band and the lateral femoral condyle as a result of rubbing as the band passes to and fro over the condyle during flexion and extension of the knee in running.

61 (a) Ecchymosis due to tracking of extravasated blood from a torn muscle.

(b) This appearance, dramatic as it may be, is nevertheless a good sign prognostically. Haematoma trapped in muscle takes far longer to settle and may leave long-term loss of extensibility.

(c) The banded appearance here is due to the fact that the patient has had his leg strapped with elastic adhesive strapping.

62 Os trigonum, or secondary ossification, representing the third or posterior malleolus on the talus. This is a congenital abnormality, usually of no significance, but entrapment may occur in activities demanding forced plantar flexion of the foot. Also demonstrated is footballer's ankle, or impingement exostosis, with projections showing on both the anterior margin of the tibia and the neck of the talus. This is *not* degenerative joint disease, as the joint gap is well-maintained.

63 A fracture and a dislocation of the head of the radius. The condition had not been diagnosed at the hospital of first presentation, and this deformity was therefore allowed to develop. Injuries in children are often difficult to diagnose, particularly when involving growing ends of bone. Re-examination and delayed radiography is frequently the key to correct diagnosis.

64 Posterior compartment syndrome. This illustrates considerable development of the deep component of the triceps surae—the soleus which is the prime mover of the ankle joint. Hypertrophy of the soleus muscle leads to increased posterior compartment pressure and avulsion of the overlying fascia from the medial tibial border.

65 This radiograph of the right ankle demonstrates clearly a thickening in the soft tissue shadow of the Achilles tendon. However, Kager's triangle between it and the structures behind the tibia is clearly defined. The lesion is therefore in the tendon alone and does not affect the paratenon. The uniformity of the lesion confirms the diagnosis— Achilles tendinitis.

66 Stress fracture of the shaft of the femur. The femur is a relatively rare site of stress fracture, but these lesions are becoming more common with the increased popularity of marathon running.

67 An excessive length of the ulnar styloid, which interferes with wrist function when the hand is held in ulnar deviation. This is a mechanical problem which can cause significant disability in racket sports and other implement sports such as hockey and lacrosse.

68 (a) Rupture of the long head of biceps brachii. The condition looks odd but it is of little, if any, clinical significance.

(b) Treatment is reassurance and continued activity to build up the remaining head of biceps and the rest of the muscles in the upper arm.

69 Myositis ossificans, or ectopic calcification in muscle. The most common site for this condition is the quadriceps mass on the front of the thigh, but it can occur in other sites. It is usually due to the compression of muscle against bone as a result of direct violence.

70 Teitze's disease. This is a peculiar inflammatory response, usually in a sternocostal rather than sternoclavicular joint, more common in women than men. It is painful but of little other significance. The aetiology is uncertain. The natural history is of spontaneous but slow remission. It may be helped by anti-inflammatory medication.

71 (a) A well-defined scoliosis of the lumbar spine made apparent by the obvious difference in contour of the flank on the right side compared with the left.
(b) This is due to protective muscle spasm which may be stimulated by, most commonly, posterior facetal joint injury or lumbar disc prolapse.

72 (a) The iliotibial band is particularly well demonstrated in this patient, who has virtually no subcutaneous fat.
(b) There is a gastrocnemius bursa present on the outer side of the popliteal fossa.

73 (a) Ectopic calcification associated, not with muscle damage as in myositis ossificans, but with joint damage. Its typical site is the elbow.
(b) During the development of the condition treatment is expectant, but once bone has formed and developed a consolidated structure the mass of ectopic ossification may be removed surgically to facilitate return to normal elbow function, as in this case.

74 This is an arthrogram of the elbow joint with the articular surfaces outlined in contrast. There is a small pouch or diverticulum from the synovial cavity on the lateral aspect of the capitellum containing a small pannus of inflamed synovial membrane.

75 (a) Loss of calcification in the carpal bones and some periarticular soft tissue thickening.
(b) The appearances are typical of hyperaemia, in this case due to infection.

76 (a) A solitary benign exostosis.
(b) It was pushing upwards under the vastus medialis and inhibiting muscle function, so leading to secondary chondromalacia patellae.
(c) Relief of symptoms and return to full normal activity was secured after a simple excision of the exostosis.

77 (a) Ectopic calcification in the supraspinatus tendon.

(b) Treatment in the acute stage is by local anaesthetic and steroid injection, or by surgical decompression of the rotator cuff and removal of the calcific deposits. In the chronic case, where pain is not extreme physiotherapy may be helpful. Many cases are found with no history of previous shoulder pain.

78 Osteosarcoma of the lower end of the femur. The radiograph shows erosion of the cortical bone and new bone deposits under the periosteum. It must always be remembered that malignant tumours and bone infection may first present as pain associated with exercise, as a result of increased tissue tension due to local hyperaemia.

79 Spondylolysis. A typical stress fracture of the pars interarticularis of L5 is shown in this oblique radiograph.

80 Cyst of the anterior horn of the medial meniscus presenting into the area of the retropatellar fat pad. The clue to diagnosis is given by the portion of meniscus clearly seen across the horizontal diameter of the specimen.

81 Avulsion of the upper attachment of rectus femoris. The presence of a well-defined epiphyseal line on the head of the femur indicates that the patient is not yet skeletally mature. Muscle avulsion strains commonly injure bone rather than soft tissue in young people.

82 Instability of the knee, with opening of the joint gap in adduction stress indicating damage to the lateral collateral ligament. When an abduction stress is applied the knee joint does not open up, indicating that the medial collateral ligament is intact.

83 (a) Avulsion fracture of the lower pole of the patella.
(b) It is usually caused by a mechanical block to forced extension of the knee, for example, the sudden stopping of the foot when tackled while attempting to kick a football.
(c) Where the displacement of the distal fragment is minimal the patient may be managed by conservative treatment with immobilisation. When there is significant displacement of the fragment it may be excised if it is small (and the defect made good) or reattached if, as in this case, it is fairly large.

84 The most likely diagnosis is stress fracture of the fibula. In this case, however, the patient was suffering from acute osteomyelitis of the lower end of the fibula. Whilst the commonest lesions present most commonly, the possibility of a more sinister cause should always be remembered and excluded.

85 Apart from a tendency for the fragments to overlap with slight shortening and/or rotation deformity of the upper arm on healing, the main complication is damage to the radial nerve in the musculospiral group. For this reason immobilisation of the fracture becomes important —if mobility is permitted at the fracture site in the early post-injury phase delayed damaged to the radial nerve may occur.

86 (a) Pelegrini–Steida disease has been thought to be ectopic calcification following avulsion injury of the medial collateral ligament, but in fact the ectopic calcification occurs proximal to its attachment.
(b) This is of little clinical significance, but it may cause pain in which case injection of local anaesthetic and steroid is helpful.

87 (a) Rupture of the ulnar collateral ligament of the first metacarpophalangeal joint (otherwise known as gamekeeper's thumb).
(b) It requires surgical repair of the ligament to restore stability in the joint. This may preclude further participation in boxing.
(c) As it is caused by inadequate closing of the hand in the glove (the boxing glove itself often prevents making a proper fist) it is prevented by making a *proper* fist inside a well-designed glove!

88 (a) Adolescent kyphoscoliosis, or Scheuermann's disease—a form of osteochondritis affecting the spine.
(b) It may be significantly exacerbated by over-energetic weight-training. It is generally advised that young athletes should not engage in training involving weights in excess of bodyweight until skeletal maturity.

89 (a) Yes.
(b) There is loss of normal contour and alignment of the vertebral bodies although no evidence of bone distortion or damage. This picture is typically seen in patients with cervical injuries, particularly posterior facetal joint problems, and is due to distortion of the normal alignment as a result of muscle spasm.

90 (a) This is an arthrogram of the ankle joint. Contrast medium is seen in the ankle joint and in the sheath of the peroneal tendons.
(b) Communication between the peroneal tendon sheaths and the ankle may be the result of complete rupture of the lateral collateral ligament of the ankle, but there may be a natural communication between these structures in a small percentage of the population.

91 (a) Displacement of the inferior humeral epiphysis. This condition may be difficult to diagnose unless radiographs of the injured elbow are taken in more than simple anteroposterior and lateral planes.
(b) The significance of this and supracondylar fracture lies, in the short term, in the risk to the artery and nerves on the anterior aspect of the elbow and, in the long term, in permanent deformity.

92 (a) Pain and tenderness over the posterior aspect of the calcaneum are typical of calcaneal apophysitis or Sever's disease. Radiographic appearances, however, are equivocal. In Sever's disease the diagnosis therefore is clinical rather than radiological.
(b) Management is by pain relief and reduction of the level of activity.

93 Valgus heels, pronating feet and chronic Achilles peritendinitis. The relationship between postural abnormality and the strains resulting therefrom with chronic overuse injury now seems clearly established. Treatment of this patient should involve postural correction of the feet by appropriate orthotics, as well as treatment of the Achilles tendon and paratenon lesions.

94 A fracture of the medial malleolus sustained some years previously with the fracture passing through the growing plate or epiphysis, leading to distortion of growth and some premature fusion. Fractures of epiphyses require close follow-up monitoring to avoid the possibility of such gross deformity developing.

95 (a) Traumatic osteolysis of the outer end of the clavicle.
(b) This usually responds to a programme of upper-body weight-training and reduction in stress from impact of tackling. In some cases, with gross secondary osteophyte formation, surgery to remove the excess bone and curette the diseased bone end may be required.

96 (a) Degenerative joint disease of the costovertebral joints. This condition is not common.
(b) The patient responded well to mobilisation and shortwave diathermy together with anti-inflammatory medication.

97 Sinding–Larsen–Johansson syndrome. This is an osteochondritis affecting the lower pole of the patella in adolescent schoolboys. It is equivalent to Osgood Schlatter's disease at the distal end of the patellar tendon, but much less common. Treatment is expectant.

98 Ultrasound scan showing psoas bursa distal to the inguinal ligament.

99 (a) Swelling on the anterior aspect of the shoulder joint over the front of the head of the humerus (the acromion process is the landmark).
(b) This is due to bicipital tendinitis with effusion in the bicipital tendon sheath.

100 Partial tear of the tibialis posterior tendon. Partial ruptures of tendons are uncommon.

101 (a) Ectopic calcification in the interosseous membrane between the tibia and fibula. It may be quite extensive and cause considerable disability. The pathogenesis of the condition is uncertain.
(b) In established cases, when the bone has become fully textured, surgical removal may be necessary and is often effective.

102 (a) Olecranon bursitis.
(b) It occurs in conjunction with friction burns in various forms of wrestling and in falls on a hard rugby or football field.
(c) It is prevented by the wearing of appropriate elasticated guards when playing on rough surfaces. Treatment is by shortwave diathermy.

103 (a) Anserine bursitis or 'breast stroker's knee'.
(b) Unco-ordinated knee action in the kick as the knees are extended and the legs brought together.
(c) Anti-inflammatory medication, shortwave diathermy and injection of local anaesthetic and steroid. Attention must be paid to swimming style.

104 Patella tendon peritendinitis. The patella tendon lies deep to the continuation of the capsule of the knee joint. Acute and later chronic inflammatory change may occur with adhesions between the deep surface of the capsule and the patella tendon, as in this case. The pathology is similar to that in Achilles peritendinitis.

105 Posterior tibial compartment syndrome, functional anterior tibial cortical hypertrophy (pretibial stress syndrome or interosseous hypertension). In some cases of stress fracture the hot node may be relatively high in the leg, but usually does not affect the whole of the tibial shadow.

106 Appearance of a bucket-handle tear of the medial meniscus through the arthroscope. These tears can frequently be removed through the arthroscope without the need for open surgery.

107 (a) Therapeutic ultrasound generator.
(b) It may be used therapeutically in the management of soft tissue injury and is also valuable in diagnosis, for example in stress fractures. In the latter case a low dose of ultrasound (less than 0.5 W/cm^2) will produce pain as the sound head is passed over the underlying stress lesion. In general ultrasound is overused in the treatment of sports injuries!

108 Stress fracture of the lower pole of the patella. It is a relatively uncommon condition. Avulsion fractures are more commonly seen, usually with separation. (The juvenile counterpart is Sinding–Larsen–Johansson syndrome.)

109 (a) Complete dislocation of the knee, in this case following a rugby accident.

(b) It is treated by reduction and surgical repair of the capsule and of the ruptured ligaments. Meniscal detachment may demand meniscectomy as well. The long-term prognosis is not good for return to sport.
(c) The most important immediate complications are damage to the popliteal vessels and/or popliteal nerve.

110 Rheumatoid arthritis—this condition is no respecter of people, even sportspeople.

111 (a) Congenital abnormality of the lumbar spine with rudimentary additional vertebra.
(b) Probably none except in an individual requiring the maximum degree of spinal joint flexibility.
(c) This patient was successfully treated by excision of the anomalous bone.

112 Osteochondritis dissecans. In this case there is a clear-cut area punched out on the lateral femoral condyle and also a small area of early osteochondritis on the medial femoral condyle.

113 (a) Spur formation with ectopic calcification in the insertion of the Achilles tendon.
(b) In persistent cases surgery may be required to excise the inevitable superficial bursa and decompress the tendon insertion, removing the ectopic bone. Conservative management is often unrewarding.

114 (a) Anterior draw sign.
(b) This is commonly thought to be due to rupture or laxity of the anterior cruciate ligament; this is only true when the anterior draw sign is elicited with the lower leg in internal rotation. In external rotation the anterior draw sign is not due to anterior cruciate damage, but to medial capsular laxity.

115 This patient has a fracture of the proximal phalanx of the little toe. No specific treatment is required other than management of symptoms. With a light spica of elastic adhesive tape and reassurance this patient was able to continue playing with no subsequent problems.

116 Stress fracture of the neck of the femur. Abnormal bone density is seen along the intertrochanteric line and the fracture can be seen on the medial border. There is some periosteal reaction on the medial side.

117 (a) Arthrogram of the wrist.
(b) Seepage of dye from the radiocarpal joint to the inferior radio-ulnar joint, indicating damage to the triangular ligament of the latter.

118 (a) This patient has a thyroid swelling, or goitre. Radiography confirmed some degree of tracheal narrowing.
(b) Surgery is indicated.

119 (a) Subluxation of the sternoclavicular joint. This condition is relatively uncommon. When it occurs it may be difficult to treat.
(b) Treatment involves anti-inflammatory medication and mobilisation of the shoulder girdle. Complete dislocation, as opposed to subluxation of the sternoclavicular joint, may cause symptoms severe enough to warrant surgical repair, but the long-term prognosis for normal function after repair is not good.

120 This patient has a secondary anserine bursitis associated with an underlying benign exostosis of the tibia. Benign exostoses are of no significance except when they cause mechanical problems, as in this case, when they may be removed.

121 Haematoma. A simple haematoma may present in a slightly unusual way and cause confusion. This is particularly true in the region of the knee, where the secondary quadriceps inhibition which results may encourage an erroneous diagnosis of internal derangement of the knee joint.

122 (a) Aspiration of a haemarthrosis.
(b) Haemarthroses should be aspirated when their presence, in terms of size and tension, is such as to interfere significantly with function of the injured joint.

123 (a) Footballer's ankle.
(b) It is not degenerative joint disease or osteoarthrosis of the ankle, since although marginal osteophytes are displayed there is no diminution of the joint gap.
(c) Treatment is expectant and conservative, except where osteophytes cause mechanical problems by impingement, then they should be removed.

124 Spondylolisthesis, forward slip of a vertebral body over that beneath it. It is caused by instability in the lumbar spine due to defects in the pars interarticularis, either as a result of stress fracture or a congenital abnormality. Spondylolysis and spondylolisthesis are relatively common findings in weight-lifters and weight-trainers (up to 20 per cent).

125 (a) Supernumerary toe.
(b) This particular patient played regular high quality football in a country where playing football barefoot was the rule. However, the laws of international football demand that in international matches football boots be worn. In order to be able to wear boots this young man needed amputation of the second toe and realignment of the first.

126 (a) Joint hypermobility (genu recurvatum). Hypermobility of joints in children, particularly when it has not been acquired by specific training, may be genuinely pathological.

(b) Children with pathological hypermobile joints should be advised against participation in body-contact sport.

127 (a) Complete rupture of the rectus femoris.

(b) The swelling demonstrated on the front of the thigh represents contracting muscle end on the proximal side of the rupture.

128 Haemarthrosis. Rapid onset swelling of the knee following injury is due to bleeding. Slow onset swelling (usually not so well marked) is due to serous effusion. Haemarthrosis denotes significant damage to soft tissues within the joint—in the knee it is usually the anterior cruciate ligament or the alar folds.

129 (a) Shortwave diathermy.

(b) Heat is generated deep in tissues by including the body in the circuit of an ultra-high frequency oscillating current. At these frequencies the heating effect of passing large currents is clinically valuable, but each pulse of current is so short that unwanted stimulation does not occur.

130 (a) Radionucleide (Technetium-99) scan demonstrating increased uptake due to inflammation in sacro-iliac joints.

(b) This appearance is diagnostic of Ankylosing Spondylitis. This case presented as low back pain in a footballer.

131 (a) Haematoma of the auricle, or 'cauliflower ear'. The skin and soft tissues are stripped from the cartilage of the ear by bleeding.

(b) Treatment is directed to replacing the soft tissues against the auricular cartilage after removal of the blood and holding them there in order for healing to take place. Too soon a return to body-contact sports invariably provokes a recurrence.

132 (a) Osgood–Schlatter's disease.

(b) It is a stress lesion of the epiphysis of the anterior tibial tubercle and may be regarded as a traction epiphysisitis. Usually it produces no problem apart from pain during the active phase and later a pronounced bony bump over the upper tibia. Occasionally the epiphysis may be avulsed.

(c) Previously management was by rest, but this is usually unnecessary; advice is to exercise within the limits of pain tolerance.

133 Early osteochondritis dissecans of the dome of the talus. A small area is well-visualised on the medial side. Treatment is expectant at this stage, with reduction of activity. Development of the condition should be monitored radiologically and it may be necessary to fix the fragment if it shows signs of separation.

134 (a) A computerised tomography (CT) scan of the calf.
(b) A translucent area deep to the shadow of gastrocnemius—this is a persistent, probably cystic, haematoma.

135 (a) Skyline radiograph showing lateral subluxation of the patella on the lateral femoral condyle.
(b) This finding is typical in patients with anterior knee pain associated with chondromalacia patellae, and is frequently due to adaptive shortening in the lateral capsule associated with vastus medialis weakness.

136 (a) Faradic stimulator.
(b) Relatively low frequency electrical pulse trains are used to stimulate the motor nerve at the motor point in normally innervated muscle to cause powerful contraction of the muscle. The feedback felt by the patient with such muscle contractions is of considerable value in restoring normal muscle control.

137 Complete rupture of the biceps femoris tendon. This is an unusual sports injury which can be managed expectantly. A repair of the biceps tendon is unnecessary.

138 A mixed lesion, showing inflamed and adherent paratenon overlying a patch of tendinitis.

139 Patella subluxation. This patient had had previous surgery to repair medial ligament damage.

140 Trigger finger. The thickened flexor tendon sheath and nodule in the tendon is clearly shown.

141 (a) Impingement exostosis on the neck of the talus.
(b) When chronically disabling, surgical excision is required.

142 (a) Arthrogram of the knee.
(b) A loose body between the patella and the femoral condyles.

143 (a) Perthe's disease, or pseudo-coxalgia. This is an epiphysitis of the upper femoral epiphysis.
(b) In severe cases it leads to distortion, premature osteoarthrosis of the hip joint and disability.
(c) Frequently as pain in the knee on exercise and it may, therefore, be overlooked. In children and adolescents the hip must always be examined as well as the knee in patients presenting with knee pain.

144 (a) Abnormal ossification of the posterior ossification centre for the talus. The usual abnormality is separation to form the os trigonum. In this

case the abnormality is fusion to the calcaneum, producing restriction of plantar flexion.
(b) Treatment is by surgical excision.

145 The calcaneal spur of itself is of no significance, but it represents the site of a traction injury where the plantar fascia is in part avulsed from the calcaneum. Cases resistant to conservative treatment including ultrasound therapy, injections and orthotic control will frequently benefit from plantar fasciotomy.

146 (a) Dislocation of the acromioclavicular joint.
(b) Wide separation of the acromion and clavicle indicates rupture of the conoid and trapezoid ligaments, requiring some form of surgical stabilisation.

147 Superficial calcaneal bursitis. This condition results from ill-fitting shoes. Immediate relief can usually be obtained by wearing a larger shoe and thick socks (better still, two or three thin socks over each other). Symptoms and swelling may also be relieved by shortwave diathermy. In chronic cases surgical excision may be required.

148 (a) Traumatic osteitis pubis. This is frequently associated with limited hip joint mobility due to slight dysplasia of the femoral head, resulting in loss of internal rotation.
(b) In the first instance anti-inflammatory medication and hip mobilising procedures should be prescribed.

149 (a) A prominent Lister's tubercle (styloid process of the second metacarpal).
(b) It sometimes produces problems of impingement in sporting activities requiring hyperextension of the wrist, e.g. shot-putting or gymnastics.

150 Epiphyseal damage in sports accidents in children may not be immediately apparent. In some instances displacement of the epiphysis may not occur immediately and radiography of the affected limb taken immediately after the accident will often show no obvious abnormality. Where severe pain following such an injury is noted, further radiographic investigation after 48–72 hours is indicated.

151 (a) Subconjunctival haemorrhages.
(b) They look dramatic but are of little clinical significance, as they resolve spontaneously leaving no long-term effects.

152 Complete rupture of the supraspinatus. This is an unusual injury, damage more commonly occurring at the tendon insertion in the rotator cuff. The loss of contour above the spine of the scapula on the left side is indicative of the diagnosis.

153 (a) Psoas bursa. Onset of symptoms in this condition is gradual and the main clinical feature is fullness in the groin and pain on exercise.
(b) Treatment is by surgical excision if disability is marked.

154 Subcutaneous haematoma. In this case the skin and subcutaneous tissues were locally avulsed from the underlying muscle fascia, with production of a large haematoma. Some days later the tracking of the extravasated blood is clearly delineated, as is the fairly localised swelling of the haematoma. A haematoma of this size will not absorb spontaneously (from this patient's leg 750 ml of blood clot was removed).

155 The patient has tenosynovitis affecting the tendons over the wrist itself (rather than proximally, as is more usual). The skin discoloration indicates that steroid injections have been given. In this case the conditon had become chronic and decompression of the extensor sheaths of the index and middle finger tendons was necessary.

156 (a) Genu varum, or bow legs.
(b) It is of no significance—many first-class athletes display a degree of bow leg. Contrast with knock-knee or valgus knee, which produces considerable problems in sportspeople.

157 (a) Avulsion of the Achilles tendon insertion in a pre-existing case of Sever's calcaneal apophysitis. The condition is rare.
(b) Treatment involves reattachment of the Achilles tendon to the posterior aspect of the calcaneum, which is technically difficult.

158 (a) Flake fracture of the tip of the lateral malleolus. Clinically these patients present with 'sprains', perhaps severe sprains.
(b) The flake fracture indicates the severity of injury but may not be apparent on initial radiography—indeed various projections may be necessary to demonstrate it. Provided that the patient is treated adequately for a lateral collateral ligament sprain, no harm is done, but too often such patients are treated inadequately, as was so in this case, so that pain and disability persist unnecessarily.

159 (a) Acetabular rim fracture as a result of overabduction and external rotation of the hip.
(b) Treatment is symptomatic when the fragment from the acetabular rim is small.

160 (a) Lumbar spondylosis with evidence of generalised disc damage.
(b) This radiograph of the spine of a rugby front row forward complaining of pain towards the end of his playing career reflects the amount of stress placed on the spine by his sport. The same type of lesion may be expected in the spine of tacklers in American football and may also be seen in competitive weight-lifters.

161 (a) Prepatellar bursitis occurs in any sport involving kneeling.
(b) When relatively small and acute it responds well to shortwave diathermy. Large, chronic examples of this type may require surgical excision, but can recur.

162 Osteochondritis dissecans. A small loose body is demonstrated in the lateral radiograph. This is a relatively common overuse injury in young sportspeople, seen particularly in gymnastics and in racket sports such as tennis. Treatment involves removal of the loose body. The outlook for the elbow is not good.

163 A cyst of the lateral meniscus. This is the classic presentation of meniscal cyst.

164 Degenerative joint disease of the distal interphalangeal joints. The typical swelling of the joints is demonstrated, and the presence of small ganglions, particularly on the index and little fingers. These should not be confused with Heberden's nodes, which are not cystic.

165 Complete rupture of the Achilles tendon. This should cause no difficulty in diagnosis. For sportspeople surgical repair offers the quickest route to return to normal function.

166 Instability of the knee due to rupture of the lateral collateral ligament. The angulation of the lower leg is clearly seen.

167 (a) A healing fracture of the middle phalanx. The line of the fracture through the joint at the base of the phalanx is clearly seen. These injuries follow a blow on the tip of the finger and are not uncommon in sports involving catching a hard or heavy ball.
(b) Management at this stage is by active use. Some degenerative joint disease in the proximal interphalangeal joint can be expected later due to involvement and distortion of the joint surface.

168 Ossifying chondroma. A relatively rare tumour, in this case lying behind the third malleolus with ectopic calcification in the lower part spreading down behind the lateral malleolus. Treatment is by simple excision of this benign lesion.

169 (a) Chondromalacia patellae. The changes on the under-surface of the patella reflect distortion in patella tracking with altered load-bearing on the articular surface.
(b) There is no correlation between the severity of damage or destruction of the articular cartilage of the patella and the patient's symptoms.

170 Typical appearance of a sprain of the lateral collateral ligament of the ankle joint. This is the commonest injury in sport—and one of the worst treated! It is not a minor injury, frequently causes considerable disability and should always be treated energetically.

171 A loose body in the intercondylar notch on tunnel view radiograph of the knee joint. A similar opacity can be seen overlying the shadow of the lateral femoral condyle. The latter is not a loose body, it is the fabella —a sesamoid in the biceps tendon.

172 (a) Acute adductor or rider's strain. This is an unusual presentation in the sense that there is an associated superficial haematoma. Usually adductor strains involve intramuscular rather than interstitial lesions.
(b) Mobilisation of the hip joint specifically to prevent scarring or adaptive shortening in the adductors.

173 Olecranon epiphysitis. Radiological appearances in this condition (which is a traction epiphysitis) are confusing: the development of ossification in the olecranon epiphysis is very variable even in the same patient and no particular appearance is diagnostic of epiphysitis.

174 (a) Degenerative joint disease of the shoulder joint. This is relatively uncommon compared with, for example, degenerative joint disease of the knee. The hatchet shape of the upper humerus is typical.
(b) The main sports injury predisposing to this lesion is recurrent dislocation of the shoulder (glenohumeral) joint.

175 (a) Ectopic calcification (myositis ossificans in the quadriceps). This is due to a direct blow on the front of the thigh.
(b) A patient presenting with such a history and marked limitation of knee flexion should be treated conservatively. Management is by shortwave diathermy and gentle active mobilisation. Other forms of treatment including vigorous massage or passive mobilisation will make the condition worse.

176 Clearly the deformity is fixed and not amenable to significant alteration. Therefore advice regarding sport should be to participate either in non-weight-bearing sports, e.g. match rifle-shooting or possibly rowing, or in static sports such as archery or trap shooting. Sports requiring high levels of mobility will probably be impossible, but simple running or jogging can be attempted given appropriate orthotic protection for the foot.

177 (a) Simple abrasion or surface burn as a result of friction between skin and, in this case, the road surface.
(b) The major problem with these lesions is secondary infection which requires appropriate preventive treatment.

178 (a) A small fracture of the margin of the proximal (talar) articular surface of the navicular.
(b) In cases of this type where symptoms are persistent, excision of the fragment gives relief.

179 (a) Asymmetry in muscle development. This appearance is common in one-handed sportspeople, particularly racket-sport players and javelin throwers. The asymmetry is to be regarded as normal. In this case some hypermobility of the right scapula is demonstrated by the extent to which it has been retracted towards the midline.
(b) The most likely diagnosis in this case is functional rhomboid pain or 'fibrositis'.

180 Degenerative joint disease of the ankle. This condition should not be confused with footballer's ankle (which also shows gross exostosis formation at the joint margins). In this case loss of normal joint space, particularly at the dome of the talus, is clearly demonstrated.

181 (a) Chronic retrocalcaneal or deep Achilles bursitis. This condition is relatively common.
(b) Conservative treatment, including local anaesthetic and steroid injections and shortwave diathermy, may be given with benefit. Once the condition becomes chronic excision of the deep calcaneal bursa is necessary for the relief of symptoms. In some cases an associated exostosis may develop on the upper posterior margin of the calcaneum, which requires removal.

182 (a) Chronic bruising due to wearing training shoes with too stiff a heel-tab.
(b) Patients with this condition are advised either to buy training shoes with no heel-tab or to remove the heel-tab from the training shoes so that pressure is not applied to the back of the heel when the foot goes into full plantar flexion.

183 (a) Focal degeneration in the Achilles tendon.
(b) The lesion, although minute, causes persistent and marked disability and illustrates the principle that the degree of disability caused by an injury is not directly related to the amount of tissue damaged.

184 (a) Avulsion injury of the hamstring from the ischial tuberosity. In young people who are not yet skeletally mature (note un-united femoral head epiphysis in this radiograph) damage to bone will often prevail over damage to related soft tissues, since the bone is still relatively soft.
(b) In this case reduction of sporting activity for a period of 3 weeks followed by progressive mobilisation would have been the treatment of choice. When the condition becomes chronic a local anaesthetic and steroid injection will often produce relief of symptoms without prejudice

to the long-term outcome, provided that the patient is discouraged from returning immediately to vigorous activity. In all cases a stretching programme must be maintained for some months.

185 (a) Acute spasmodic torticollis.
(b) Analgesics and the provision of a close-fitting collar may be adequate, but the patient should be closely watched in the first few days following the injury, and if the spasm persists gentle mobilisation under general anaesthetic will restore normal alignment and movement in the cervical spine. Following this procedure return to sport should be delayed while the patient undergoes a programme of stretching and mobilising exercises.

186 In clinical terms very little! This is a benign exostosis on the upper humerus of no functional significance. However, (i) it does illustrate the extent to which irrelevant clinical abnormalities may present in association with sports trauma and (ii) it is a reminder of the need to follow up and investigate such abnormalities and to bear in mind the possibility that they may be of real clinical significance, e.g. that the lesion may be malignant rather than benign.

187 (a) Multiple calcifying loose bodies from synovial chondromatosis.
(b) Treatment is by removal.
(c) Remarkably good.

188 (a) Gross thickening and scarring in the Achilles paratenon.
(b) Surgery of the Achilles tendon itself for overuse injury, unless accompanied by the removal of the paratenon from the insertion on the calcaneum to the musculotendinous junction, will almost invariably result in a recurrence of symptoms due to subsequent secondary scarring in the paratenon.

189 (a) Swelling over the lower lumbar spine may be associated with congenital abnormalities of the spina bifida type. When these are marked, neurological changes are present in the lower limbs, causing a greater or lesser degree of disability. Such conditions are, however, rare in active sportspeople.
(b) It is unlikely that a swelling of this size would be associated with a spina bifida. In fact, this was a simple lipoma.

190 (a) This patient has cellulitis as a secondary complication of a haematoma of the skin and subcutaneous tissues. This site over the front of the tibia is particularly prone to such an injury or to deeper subperiosteal haematoma.
(b) In this case treatment with antibiotics and rest to extinguish the infection is all that is required.

191 (a) Complete rupture of the lateral collateral ligament of the ankle. In this case the excessive inversion and the prominence of the lateral malleolus give the clue to the diagnosis.

(b) Chronic lateral ligament injuries of the ankle may show complete rupture, as in this case, where the patient complains of instability and talar tilt is demonstrated radiologically on stress radiography.

192 Sebacious cyst. This is not a usual site for a sebacious cyst, and the case illustrates the point that it is necessary always to be alert for conditions presenting in an unusual manner or place.

193 Thoracic inlet syndrome. There are prominent transverse processes of C6 and rudimentary cervical ribs on C7. When there is significant interference with function, exploration and removal of the rib or fibrous band must be carried out.

194 Subluxation of the acromioclavicular joint with fractures of the outer end of the clavicle. Note that the acromioclavicular joint gap here is not so wide as to indicate disruption of the conoid and trapezoid ligaments.

195 (a) Hallux rigidus, or degenerative joint disease affecting the first metatarsophalangeal joint.

(b) Conservative treatment includes the provision of a stiff sole or metatarsal rocker, or manipulation under general anaesthetic with injection of the joint using local anaesthetic and steroid. In chronic cases arthroplasty or arthrodesis may be required.

(c) Excision arthroplasty in a patient with Morton's foot (long second toe) leads to mechanical problems unless a spacer is used.

196 (a) The radiograph shows fracture of the neck of the radius, distal to the upper radial epyphysis. The fracture line goes through the epiphyseal line.

(b) Conservative management with gentle mobilisation is the initial treatment. This patient must be followed up to monitor the progress of development of the proximal end of the radius.

197 The photograph illustrates the rehabilitation of the extensor muscles of the knee using the De Lorme boot. This method of rehabilitation is physiologically unsound, since the weight of the boot distracts the knee joint surfaces, whereas under normal conditions and loading the knee joint surfaces are compressed.

198 Low-grade chronic osteomyelitis. Osteomyelitis usually presents in the acute phase but may develop insidiously, as in this case, and cause problems in diagnosis. This patient's white cell count was normal, as was the sedimentation rate, but there was greatly increased uptake of radionucleide on bone scanning.

199 (a) Fracture of the malar bone with obvious depression of the cheek.

(b) Complications include diplopia due to distortion of the inferior margin of the orbit, anaesthesia of the cheek due to possible damage to the infraorbital nerve and osteomyelitis if fracture opens into an infected sinus.

200 (a) Patient has a 'black eye', or periorbital haematoma.

(b) Because of the nature of the injury there may be damage to any of the structures of the globe.

(c) Early examination of the patient involves gentle opening of the eyelids to check the patient's sight; if there is any doubt, the patient should be referred for a specialist ophthalmalogical opinion. Ocular damage to the eye occurs with monotonous regularity in certain ball games, particularly squash rackets, and also in some body-contact sports. Where possible, preventive goggles or glasses should be worn.

Postscript

While it is generally true that clear patterns of injury emerge for different sports, reflecting the type and manner of stresses on and in the body developed in that sport, there remains nevertheless a great deal of opportunity for the unexpected, the unlikely and the rare to present. Sometimes the clinical features of the case, either the history or the findings on clinical examination, or the results of specialist investigation are clear-cut but often they are not. Diagnosis is only half the battle in the management of injury but accurate diagnosis is the foundation, and the only effective foundation, for logical management thereafter. The demands of the sportsman for effective treatment are inevitably more strident and more pressing than those of the ordinary man in the street. Inevitably the satisfying of such demands is of itself a source of immense satisfaction.